Detoured Destiny

One Woman's Road to Recovery

Jessica M. Davenport

Detoured Destiny

Copyright © 2018 by Jessica M. Davenport

All rights reserved. No part of this book may be reproduced or transmitted in any form or by any means without written permission from the author. Some characters have been renamed and some identifying details changed to protect the privacy of individuals.
ISBN (978-1986650977)

ISBN (1986650979)

Printed in the USA by CreateSpace.com (www.createspace.com)

This book is dedicated to the hundreds of girls and women
whose candles blew out too soon
when they died following complications with birth control.

Table of Contents

Acknowledgements 6

1. Girl Meets World 7
2. Vertigo 9
3. I Feel Pretty 12
4. Here Comes the Boom 17
5. All in the Family 20
6. ER 27
7. Friends 33
8. Coma 40
9. Big 48
10. School's Out 53
11. Up 57
12. The Perfect Storm 59
13. Accepted 61
14. Supernatural 71

15	Funny Girl	73
16	17 Again	78
17	The Ugly Truth	82
18	Home Is Where the Heart Is	89
19	What Lies Beneath	93
20	Kids Say the Darnedest Things	97
21	Grownups	103
22	To Hell and Back	107
23	A Walk to Remember	112
24	Love and Marriage	116
25	Back to School	122
26	Easy A	124
27	A Fork in the Road	128
	Notes	132
	Bibliography	136

Acknowledgements

I want to thank my family and friends for giving me the courage and help to write about my experience and publish this book. Especially Mom, Aunt Kristen Falcone, Aunt Chris Johnson, Uncle Mark Davenport, Uncle Brian Falcone, Uncle Carl Johnson, and all my cousins (particularly David McReynolds, Kyle Hefton, Isabella Falcone, Olivia Falcone), thank you for donating and helping with fundraising.

I didn't think anyone needed to know my story and thought few other people were afflicted with my blood disorder. But then my former high school English teacher, Ms. Foster, got me in contact with a girl whose sister died from the same blood disorder and stroke and, wait for it, she went to the same high school as me and she died after my accident. I could have warned her and thousands of other girls about the possible dangers.

After that I went to my friend Nataja and said, "Okay, book time." She had hounded me for a while to tell my story. Nataja Wells, I can't thank you enough for your help. I love you and you're my you-know-what! I also thank my editor, Susan Robinson, for encouraging me to discuss even uncomfortable subjects and for her ability to pull so much out of me.

Hopefully you all love this book as much as I do!

1
Girl Meets World

At nineteen, I suffered a stroke. Plunged into a coma, I floated, Mom's sobs and my brother's scent swirling as I awaited true love's kiss and happily ever after. Instead I awoke to a woman in blue scrubs holding my hand. She explained that I would never use my arms or legs or speak again. The worst part was that none of it had to happen. But no one warned me.

I was a smoker and unaware I had a blood disorder. Adding birth control to the mix hit the trifecta—the combination created a clot that cut off blood flow to an area in my brain. Seriously? Birth control is supposed to prevent a drastic event from happening in your life, not trigger one. Who would believe my stroke might have been caused by a combination of things including my birth control?

After years of saying no and finding reasons why I shouldn't, I'm ready, or as ready as I'll ever be, to tell my story. The truth is, I feel a downright responsibility to tell my story to women everywhere. I'd feel mighty selfish hanging onto this information. By telling my story, I hope to prevent a repetition of it. All women considering birth control need to know its dangers. Everyone should take precautions to prevent a life-shattering event. Sure, you read the package's warnings and side effects and think none of them will happen to you. I thought that too, but am living proof that they can. Please talk to your doctor or healthcare professional and get all the facts before you start birth control.

With that said, I wouldn't change what happened to me. The sayings, "You don't know how strong you are until the shit hits the fan" and "God wouldn't bring you to it if He couldn't pull you through it" have real meaning now. Surviving a stroke matured me so much. I'd never want my life to go back to the way it was before. Believe it or not, I recognize the value of what happened to me and I'm okay with it! At first it seriously challenged me, though. Every day I prayed for the sweet relief of death. Control was—is—my middle name; I planned nosebleeds. This was not in my plans!

I seldom plan anymore. While writing an excerpt for this book, I had an epiphany about my tattoos. It's hard to believe it's taken me this long to see the connection. Two tattoos I got at the age of eighteen were both unplanned and spur of the moment. The first, a cute butterfly on my foot, was inked February 17, 2001; the second, a four-leaf clover that says "Lucky," was added on my hip June 17, 2001.

My butterfly tattoo now seems a perfect symbol of my rebirth. The former teenaged and tarnished me cocooned, crystalized, and emerged a butterfly—a mature and caring woman who enjoys learning as much as teaching.

As for that little shamrock on my hip, what started as a joke to my friends and me when I first got it has come to mean so much more to me now. I am Lucky to be alive, and the shamrock's shade of green is the color for my blog! And now for the kicker: my stroke was March 17, 2004. Everything happened on the 17th!

After a lifetime of planning everything, I've found that the things that mean the most to me now are those I didn't plan. I guess it's true what they say—you make plans and God laughs!

2
Vertigo

Did you ever just know there was something really bad wrong with you?

The night of March 16, 2004 started out perfectly normal. My best friend, Trav, and our bud George lounged on the couch at my house. Smoking a cigarette, I hunched over the coffee table as I drew a map for my little brother, Blake's, homework assignment. Even though I wasn't the best artist, I ordinarily drew his maps for school and he colored them.

Our miniature Yorkie, Harley, stepped around the pillows and blankets strewn all over the floor, hopped into my lap, and went limp.

I put out my cigarette. "What is wrong with you?" I asked, picking up the six-pound ball of fluff and staring into his eyes. Although Harley was technically Blake's dog, I took the most care of him. He licked my face; I put him down and continued outlining Brazil.

Harley jumped back up into my lap and again poufed himself like a powder puff.

"Huh?" I cuddled him, then put him down.

Twice more, Harley flopped into my lap. Blake and I checked him over and couldn't find anything wrong with him.

"He's just an attention whore," Blake said. He held the dog, so I could finish adding the Amazon River.

They say dogs know sometimes, and he knew.

After Trav and George left around eleven, Blake and I went to Wal-Mart to buy *The Blue Collar Comedy Tour* DVD (the first one). Up in college I had seen it and thought it was hilarious! As we walked out of Wal-Mart, I started to feel light-headed.

"Do you feel dizzy?" I asked Blake.

When he answered, "Yes," I became worried for both of us. I was afraid we had inhaled gas. But as we pulled into our driveway he started laughing and said, "I'm just kidding, Sissy. I don't feel dizzy."

I yelled, "Dammit, Blake! I don't feel good and you're bullshitting me!"

My parents were in the kitchen. I told Dad I felt dizzy.

"Is it your regular carsick dizzy?"

I nodded.

"Take your Dramamine. Do you have it?"

I kept the medicine in my purse because I always got carsick, and it helps with motion sickness. I hadn't taken it when I first felt sick at Wal-Mart because I was under the impression that my brother felt dizzy too.

After I popped the pills, Blake, Mom, and I went up to my room to watch the movie. They loved it! Focused on the movie, I didn't notice my dizziness so much.

After the movie, Mom and Blake went downstairs to bed, but I couldn't sleep. My head still felt woozy, and I was consumed with this horrible feeling in the pit of my stomach that something was wrong or something really bad was going to happen to me. I can't even describe the feeling, but if you have felt it, you'd know. At first I didn't tell anybody because I thought I was being paranoid, but eventually I called my ex, Samuel (my longest relationship—two months), and my friend Nathan. Neither answered, but I left messages as I cried and told their voice mail, "I feel like something's wrong with me and need to talk to somebody."

After I called them both, I lay in bed awhile and tried to relax. Around four a.m., still feeling dizzy and strange, I went downstairs to ask Mom to come upstairs. Whenever I felt sick I always asked Mom to come sleep next to me—call me a big kid. One of the worst feelings to have is an instinct that something is wrong but not knowing or being able to piece together what it is, almost as if fingers from another realm of consciousness are poking into your brain.

Remember the serial killer on *Dexter* who convinced the woman to commit suicide? He whispered in my ear, "Everything's fine. You're just paranoid. Shhh…go to sleep. Everything will be back to normal tomorrow."

That night I experienced the true power of fear, and I don't spook easily.

3
I Feel Pretty

Who is Jessica Davenport? Well, that depends on whether you are talking to the nineteen-year-old "southern princess" or my more mature and empathetic thirty-something self. Labeling myself a "southern princess" sounds ridiculous to me now. Then, it just meant I considered myself a small-town southern girl in a well-to-do family. Pre-stroke, if I had to sum myself up in three words they would have been perfectionist, people-pleaser, and personable. To this day I have to admit there is still a bit of truth to the perfectionist and the people-pleaser, but I am not especially personable any more.

Before my stroke my room and bathroom stayed organized and color-coded. My friends asked me over to organize their closets. Now that I can't use my hands great, seeing a crooked picture frame is frustrating and having a V-neck shirt not centered on my chest bugs the shit out of me. I ask to have them adjusted. I must have things my way and just right or it drives me nuts! Frequently I ask my aide or Mom to put everything in my closet in certain baskets and label them. If they get disorganized I sometimes go *Silence of the Lambs* on people and scream, "Put the lotion in the flippin' basket!" But because I am pestered by the need to please others, I yell with a smile. If someone doesn't get a kick out of me, I bug them until we're friends. It's sad, but true. Isn't everybody a people-pleaser to some degree? Please tell me I don't stand alone. I used to love to interact with and introduce myself to new people. Now I feel uncomfortable around most new people.

This is not how I saw my life playing out. My dream was to be a stay-at-home mom: meet my husband in college, get married, and have four or five kids. Typical southern girl existence. I would never have guessed that at the age of thirty-three this is where life would have taken me. A mute quadriplegic. This is so not a life I would have chosen for myself. Would anyone?

Now my life consists of wheelchairs and lifts and physical, occupational, and speech therapy. My days are filled with learning how to express my feelings and emotions in this "new" body and having to listen to the mwa-mwa-mwa of doctors and nurses and therapists all with their own ideas of who I am and what I'm capable of physically and emotionally. A couple of years ago I had a little accident (well, not so little—I tumbled down eight steps in my chair) and messed up my back. The pain was *extreme*. My aides told me they knew I was suffering when my face got red and I held my breath. Since most of my day is spent sitting in a chair, the condition is degenerating, and it still hurts like a bitch sometimes. I am sensitive as well to other painful back and stomach sensations.

Before my stroke I dealt with bad period cramps; now they hurt *so* much worse. Along with these I sometimes get ovarian cysts. Some people don't even know they have cysts, but I can tell whether mine is on the left or right ovary. When one bursts I often pass out or throw up from the pain.

My life is no longer my own, and I fear that's a wound not even time can heal. The few moments I get to sit quietly are treasures. I no longer get to keep much to myself. Internally I can hold secrets, but externally my life's an open book. Over the years, I have grown somewhat okay with openness (as you will read in this book), but for heaven's sake give me some damn dignity! For example, before my stroke, if someone walked into the room while I was getting dressed, I could quickly grab a shirt to cover me. Now, if my aides are doing my care and someone walks in while I'm naked, I am lucky to get covered. Everybody just gets a free peep show—minus the pole.

The past several years I've struggled to balance the progress I've made physically and emotionally with the need to stay encouraged despite the length of the process. Some people don't think I have it in me to get back to who I was before the wheelchair, and I want to be able to yell, "I told you so!" Getting back even a fragment of my former self would be nice. I don't require the whole package—I want the strong, youthful body, but not the selfish, immature mind.

Often, I mention that I remain thankful for what happened to me because in a strange way it *saved my life*. It truly did. I'd never go back to the girl I was before the stroke—the girl who used alcohol, drugs, and sex to mask her emotions. Alcohol, especially, was becoming a good friend. I could get drunk and act stupid and not tell people my feelings. I am much more content with getting to know the woman I have become and grooming the woman I am soon to be. All the maturity and spiritual growth I gained I owe to the many adversities I faced. I feel much more woke and empathetic than I used to, and only some of it is because of age. The rest I attribute to my traumatic experience and the religious growth it triggered. Without the obstacles there'd be no me. Although I still cuss like a sailor and talk about really inappropriate things sometimes (as you will read in this book), my relationship with the Man upstairs gets a little stronger each day.

To add to my teenaged need for perfection and masks, I had become bulimic. So ironically, the stroke kept me from screwing up my life. I imagine God looking down at me and shaking His head, saying, "That's not a good path, Jessica. Where's the reset button?"

    In my stereotypical small southern hometown, everyone goes to the high school football game on Friday night and church Sunday morning, and everyone is in *everyone's* business. It's so bad that I emailed a hello to Jonah, a friend I hadn't talked to since high school, and he knew exactly how my stroke occurred! "How did you know?" I wrote, and he replied, "Small town."

    Even though Jonah was right about what happened to me, a lot of other people from my hometown know only the "telephone game" version. They have the kernel of the story, but the details are a little bit off. I have heard some doozies over the years. Let's see: I developed a brain tumor, I had a brain aneurysm that burst, or Dad gave me experimental medicine and it went bad. Let's dissect these incorrect assumptions. The brain is the correct area of my body affected. You most likely die from brain tumors and burst aneurysms, so if I had died you would have been almost right. The experimental medicine rumor gets a round of applause for literally making my family and me laugh out loud. Experimental medicine, seriously? Yeah, Dad's a doctor, but there's a minute chance that he could have gotten his hands on experimental medicine and then given said medicine to his child. Putting my smart-ass attitude aside, at least these jokers are "trying" to understand it. You want the true story, please just ask me.

Thankfully, Jessica Davenport has grown up and matured over the years. But I wouldn't be me without my past.

4
Here Comes the Boom

You never wake up and realize it's the last day of your life. Open your eyes and think, I'll never pick up Bre for school again, never again make scrambled eggs with a gallon of ketchup for breakfast with Blake.

Frankly, it never crosses your mind. We all know we aren't promised tomorrow, but that never stops us from setting out our clothes for the next morning or making dinner plans for that night with friends. There's this little part in all of us that makes us feel invincible. We know bad things happen to people, just not to us. Although occasionally we're wrong. *Man, oh man, was I wrong.*

After Mom came upstairs with me I finally fell asleep, but woke when she got up at six the next morning to get ready for work as an ultrasound technician. I clumped downstairs to tell her bye and that I still didn't feel well. She begged me to stay home and rest. Listening to her plea, I went back upstairs to lie down after she left.

Mom and I even remember me going up the stairs doing my usual one, two, skip-a-few climb.

Once I got back to my room, I couldn't sleep because I kept needing to pee. As time went on I grew dizzier and dizzier, and I just had this insistent gut feeling that something was off.

Finally I went downstairs to get Dad to come and lie with me. For this Momma's girl to seek out Dad because I didn't feel well was big. He knew that it meant I felt tremendously sick. As soon as we lay down I needed to pee again. I walked back to the bathroom and fell about ten feet from the doorway.

Dad ran to help me up. "What happened, Sis?"

"I'm f-f-fine. I just f-fell w-walking to the b-bathroom, b-but I landed on my b-butt."

As a former ER doctor Dad had seen a lot of patients with head trauma, so he had taught my brother and me that any time we fell we should try to sit: "A broken tailbone is easier to fix than a broken head." During his residency and for several years after he worked in the ER, that knowledge had come in handy.

His training kicked in and he started asking me questions as he noticed my speech continue to slur.

"What are you doing today?"

"C-cleaning and m-m-meeting Trav and then p-picking up B-B-Blake from s-s-school."

"Do you know the weather? I didn't hear it."

"I-I think i-i-it's g-going to be n-n-nice."

Dad knew something was wrong with me, but he didn't know what. My mom had done ultrasound for many years and had lots of medical knowledge, and he knew she knew her shit, so he called her. "Listen to Jessica," he said, putting the phone in my face.

I remember trying to tell Mom, "I need to go to the hospital. I can't talk right," but my speech slurred so much it came out, "Hos-s-split-tal." It felt like I had a mouth full of marbles.

Mom yelled, "What's wrong with you? What's wrong with you?"

Dad walked to my door and said, "Get dressed. We're going to the hospital."

On the other side of the door, Dad hissed at the phone. "Get home NOW! She's deteriorating too fast for an ambulance!" They both believed it looked neurological but thought, *It can't be a stroke—she's too healthy and young.*

My dad went downstairs to let us both get dressed. I felt like I was drunk, stumbling around to get my shorts off and pants on. Although she worked twenty minutes away, Mom rushed into my room in a flash to help me pull on my sweatshirt and shoes. Relief fell over me. We stumbled downstairs and she and dad walked me to Mom's car. I lay in the backseat. We all rushed to the hospital where Mom worked.

I even remember the outfit I threw on for the hospital: my maroon Gap sweatshirt, blue American Eagle pants (with paint on the butt), and multi-color tennis shoes.

I would never take the stairs one, two, skip-a-few to my bedroom again. There would be no more making breakfast with Blake.

5
All in the Family

I grew up in the "perfect" American family—dad, mom, two kids, and a dog. However, since I was adopted by Dad, he's technically my stepfather.

My biological father is from Costa Rica. He and Mom's brother were college roommates. He traveled often for work, leaving Mom and me home together a lot. They divorced when I was one and he moved back to Costa Rica.

Over the years my biological father and I have talked some. At sixteen, I flew to Costa Rica by myself to meet him. He and I had wanted me to come alone, but in reality, I needed Mom. It was a confusing and uncomfortable trip. I called and emailed my friend Savi and Mom, crying my eyes out.

"I don't know these people," I said, "and they're my family."

I know little about my biological father, so little that a couple of years ago, Mom and I got into an argument about my heritage. She told someone I was part Italian, and I was mad she lied—only to find out that my biological father *is* of Italian heritage. Maybe I had better order that kit from ancestry.com—because it's sad not knowing.

Anyway, my stepfather raised me, so he's Dad. I figured I'd clear that up before we got any farther.

One awesome point about Dad is, in the thirty-ish years he's existed in my life, *he never once uttered the words, "You aren't my daughter." He always tells me he married Mom because of me.*

My parents met through a lady at work. Mom is from Pennsylvania but moved to Tennessee (where I was born) for my biological dad's job; during the divorce we moved back to Pennsylvania.

A lady at the hospital where they both worked told Mom, "You should meet this great guy in residency. And he's from Tennessee!"

My mom straightaway thought, *Ugh, no more Tennessee.* Then she met Dad and the rest is history.

We do, however, enjoy teasing Dad about the way he asked Mom for their first date: "Me and some friends are going to the movies. You can come if you want." Smooth, Dad. Real smooth.

My dad was a total bachelor in his mid-thirties when he and Mom dated. He had never been around many children but was a big kid himself, and he and I instantly clicked. I couldn't say his name and called him "Rathy." They both laugh about trying to teach two-year-old me to say Larry: "La La La-r-ry…La-Rathy!"

One time when they were dating, Mom had to work and couldn't find a babysitter for me, so Dad offered. She dropped my diaper bag and me off at his apartment and went to work. Apparently I pooped an explosion while there. He started to change me, but Mom hadn't packed enough wipes. Holding me upside down by the feet (like a turkey) in the shower, Dad decided to let the water rinse my butt. Just as he lifted my feet, Mom walked in and screamed,

"What are you doing?! The shit's gonna rinse in her face!" I just laughed hysterically about our new game.

Blake came into this world when I turned six, and I told my parents adamantly, "You can be the first ones to hold him in the delivery room, but I am the first person to kiss him." That fondness faded when I realized I wasn't the baby any more (thankfully, that jealousy lasted all but five minutes).

Granny (Mom's mom) said I told her right after Blake was born, "I didn't like him at first, but I love him now!"

Blake and I didn't fight much (I hear from other people how much they fought with their siblings), and if we did it was usually because we were teasing each other about something. He had this thing about people showing skin. No one else could show skin, but he stayed naked the first ten years of life. Teasing him about it was my favorite pastime. Remember the song by Petey Pablo that says, "Take your shirt off and swing it around like a helicopter"? Every time we heard it we danced. I teased him: "Look, I do this at the club (bar)." Then I lifted my shirt up to show my stomach.

Blake yanked down my shirt and yelled, "Quit it, Sissy! Mom! Sissy's taking her shirt off *in public*!" In the club I did pull my shirt up, but much less than I did in front of Blake.

Older sisters will agree with me that little brothers sometimes say embarrassing things. One time while I was getting ready to go to the club, my brother, in front of my boyfriend, pointed to the stretch marks on my hips. "What's that?" he said. Embarrassed that he had pointed out an unbecoming flaw, I punched him in the arm.

Blake and I stayed close growing up, but we became two peas in a pod after I graduated high school. I took him to every baseball practice and game and picked him and his friends up from school every day. On his birthday I surprised him and checked him out of school—you know, typical big sister stuff.

Blake, Dad, and Mom always call me "Sis" or "Sissy." Even some of Blake's friends call me "Sis."

Until he was twelve or thirteen, Blake slept in my parents' room every night, except the nights he slept in my room. When he was little, Mom accidentally traumatized him with a story about a little girl who was kidnapped through the window of her ground floor bedroom—and he had a ground floor bedroom.

Every Christmas Eve, Blake stayed in my room, and after a sleepless night we used our house's intercom system to wake our parents around six a.m. (our parents are *not* morning people, so the early wake up took a while). After Dad's brother and their parents (my uncle doesn't have children, so Blake and I are the only grandkids on that side) arrived, Dad covered our eyes and led us downstairs. Going down the steps with your eyes closed is intimidating, so I always grabbed on tight to Dad's arm to keep from falling. Once we reached the bottom and entered the living room, he uncovered our eyes and everybody yelled, "Merry Christmas!" Blake and I gasped and ran to our separate piles—Santa always separated our presents so they were easier to pick through.

Watching tons of movies multiple times was a favorite family pastime. Throughout this book you will discover a plethora of movie quotes. Even now we email and text each other random movie quotes. Sorry to say though, most of the movies are old, as our parents corrupted us on eighties and nineties movies. Blake does a spot-on impression of the car scene in the movie *Weird Science*. It's hilarious!

When we weren't watching movies, the hub of our house was the kitchen. A huge center island contained the stove and a dinner table. We all cooked everything, but my passion is baking desserts. My friends at school always asked me to bring cakes and cookies.

On some weekends Mom used to do this thing with me she called "midnight snack." She would bring a tray to my room with saltines, cheese, and mustard to make sandwiches. I miss our midnight snacks. It's not that easy anymore to bring me food late at night.

My mom is an ultrasound technician and Dad is a family practice doctor. For approximately fourteen years he had a medical practice in a popular tourist town forty-five minutes away from our home. The office stayed busy for many years. Ours was a comfortable life and we knew it. Four bedrooms and a bonus room were more than enough for the four of us. We loved our home and were happy. When we first bought it Dad would joke with people who called, answering the phone in an English accent: "Hellew. Davenport residence. This is the butlaaaar."

My friends and I spent summers splashing in our pool, judging who did the best dive or who could hold their breath the longest for underwater laps. Wintry weekend evenings found us lounging in the hot tub. We used to bet on who could stand in the snow the longest before scooting into the hot tub (we used to bet one another often for any inane reason). The gym and office, however, stayed brand spanking new. In high school I convinced my parents to let me convert the bonus room into my boudoir. I painted the walls a purplish blue, moved around furniture, and bought a comforter that matched.

The office's outside door opened to the bottom driveway (we had two). Mom sometimes sequestered herself in the office paying bills or something, leaving the door open to watch Blake, our two friends Kipp and Kory, and me playing. After Blake was born, my parents used to bicycle a lot. They towed Blake and me in a little yellow cart that Blake and I played with when we got older.

One afternoon, Kipp, Kory, Blake, and I tried to see who could ride their bike the fastest with somebody in the cart. It was my turn to ride in the cart, and I brought chips and a plastic cup of Sprite. Kipp drove, speeding down the driveway, but he didn't see a little rock in our path. The cart hit the rock and flipped in the air. I flew out, still holding the drink, and hit the concrete driveway. The drink pooled around me as I lay face down, motionless. Hearing the crash, Mom looked up. From inside the office several feet away, she thought the drink pooling around me was blood. She screamed and ran to me, then realized the pool wasn't blood. I was fine, only suffering a few scratches. We still tease Mom for mistaking soda for blood.

    Turns out Mom's sixth sense about me wasn't so bad after all…not that anyone would listen.

6
ER

Mom sped on the highway, delivering me to the hospital in fifteen minutes. My memory after getting there is shit, so I only remember little snippets. By then I could barely walk, so my parents helped me into a wheelchair. Dad had driven separately to the ER ahead of us to warn them about my ever-worsening condition. He told the admitting nurse that it looked like I was having a stroke or some other neurological event. Her response was, "If there's no family history of strokes that's probably not it." They made me wait.

Finally I was examined to try to determine a diagnosis. Everyone was trying to figure out what was happening to me. Ethically, doctors aren't allowed to treat themselves or family members, so Dad had to stand back and watch them treat me. He said later that it felt unbearable for him.

I heard someone mention meningitis and someone else suggest I could have West Nile virus. To rule out the possibility of an infectious disease they tested my white blood cell count. A high count might mean an infection. Much to their surprise, my white blood cell count tested normal.

Nobody thought "stroke." Strokes happen to elderly people, not teenagers. Even so, they checked my brain with a computerized tomography (CT) scan. According to the Mayo Clinic, a CT scan "combines a series of x-ray images taken from different angles and uses computer processing to create cross-sectional images, or slices, of the bones, blood vessels and soft tissues inside your body."[1]

Trav was there when the technician was just about to do my CT Scan. He and Mom warned him I'm scared of small spaces, but I don't think anyone realized just how claustrophobic. The technician gave me Valium, but it didn't work, so he put a button in my hand and said, "Push this if you get nervous, and we'll stop." As soon as he slid me into the tube for the scan I hit the button. I remember him sounding almost annoyed over the intercom: "Okay, Ms. Davenport, you're going to have to stay in longer than that." Mom had to put on a lead apron to protect her from radiation while she stood beside the scanner and held my hands. Even though my CT appeared negative for stroke and "unremarkable" (according to my hospital records), my parents still thought that stroke remained a possibility.

You can't wear metal in the machine, and I had a belly button ring. Afterward, Mom disclosed that it was hard to get out. She kept shaking, and they were rushing her. The ring had an angel on one end and a devil on the other.

After my blood tests came back normal, the doctors consulted a neurologist. "Finally!" my parents said. They had been screaming it was neurological from the beginning.

Once the neurologist arrived (thirty to forty-five minutes later) he did sternum rubs on me and I got so annoyed. For those of you who don't know, sternum rubs are when they rub the bone in your chest with the palm of their hand. The point is to wake you up. Part of me knew what he was doing, and the other part of me didn't and thought he was trying to cop a feel. He kept rubbing, and I kept smacking his hand, scoffing at him and saying to myself, *Dude! Enough—quit it!* Thinking back, I realize he was probably as annoyed as I was.

My speech became progressively worse as I went from slurring my sentences to mumbling two words to being unable to speak, but I wanted to scream, "Quit with the damn tests! Everybody needs to leave me the hell alone and let me sleep!" I remember Mom taking my cell phone to call some of my friends. Bre was at school two hours away, but Trav and Savi came straight to the hospital. Trav came to my bedside without delay while Savi stayed in the waiting room. Unable to talk at all, I couldn't stop shaking. I could only write "I love you" on a piece of paper. Although Trav and I considered ourselves just best friends, we said "I love you" constantly. Honestly, we had both developed feelings for each other, but I was scared if we broke up it would ruin the friendship.

Looking back, I should have written that note to my parents too, but they knew I loved them.

I recall looking around and it was like a movie—everybody was in fast motion, except I was in slow motion. If you've ever studied dissociative disorders, it felt comparable to that. Some degrees of the disorder make people feel almost outside of their bodies watching the traumatic events they're experiencing. Everything was just going so fast I wasn't scared by what was happening to me; I was a spectator. There was just a shrug of the shoulders and a glib feeling of thinking, *Ehh, what happens, happens.*

At one point, I remember doctors doing a lumbar puncture (LP). Also known as a spinal tap, an LP is a diagnostic and/or therapeutic procedure in which a doctor collects cerebrospinal fluid for laboratory analysis.[2] The test requires you to lean forward, and I could barely hold myself up. Dad sat in front of me, and I felt so exhausted I just laid my head on his shoulder and fell asleep. I am told an LP is painful, and the fact that I slept through it should have told my doctors that something affected my pain tolerance. One of the functions of the reticular formation in the brain (which was near where my stroke occurred) has to do with pain leniency (BTW I still possess a high pain tolerance!).

If the fluid withdrawn on a spinal tap happens to be cloudy or colored that means the patient might have an infection or disease. Dad argued with the doctor: "Her white blood cells are normal and her spinal tap was clear. She does not have an infection. It's neurological!"

The doctor answered: "Your daughter is dying and we don't know why!"

Because my initial CT appeared clear, they put all their eggs in the encephalitis (viral infection) basket and didn't agree with Dad. Most people my age with similar symptoms suffer from a type of encephalitis. Plus, West Nile Virus was new then and not seen often.

My parents later told me that I kept snoring while I slept in the ER, which is weird because I had never snored.

Many years of speech therapy tell me that should have been a clue to my doctors. My throat muscles were weakening and doctors probably needed to intubate me instead of making the sudden decision to give me a tracheostomy, a hole in my neck to breathe.

I don't personally hold this next memory, but every time Mom tells this story it makes me cry. When Mom told Blake they didn't know what was wrong with me and he overheard the doctor say I might die, he ran out of the ER and across the street. When she caught up to him, tears welled up in his big brown eyes.

"That is my only sister and I can't lose her," Blake said. (I know you're crying. I am too!) That's hard news for anyone, but no thirteen-year-old should have to hear that and face the mortality of a sibling. It always eats me up.

Once they finally listened to Mom's "stroke!" screams, doctors asked me to sit up and smile. A distorted smile is a marker for a stroke, and they wanted to check mine. It took so long because stroke wasn't on their radar. They kept telling themselves, *It can't be a stroke; it must be something else.* Even when they checked my smile, the doctors debated whether it looked crooked.

Mom stood behind them, arms crossed. "I have seen that smile for nineteen years," she said. "That's not it."

The last thing I remember from that day is sitting up in bed in my hospital room, where they had moved me after the ER. I was laughing with Bre and her mom and some other people, and then they left to go to the hospital cafeteria. Suddenly I couldn't breathe and nurses came running into my room. Then everything went black. Doesn't that just sound like a typical *Lifetime* movie scene?

You know how people sometimes get remarkably better before dying? Maybe sitting up, talking without slurred speech, and joking was my remarkable event. Maybe I was supposed to die, but God changed His mind. Hmmm.

The next morning, March 18th, they gave me another CT scan and it showed "some decreased attenuation of the central pons," which is a fancy phrase saying that the blood flow to part of my brain stem slowed. Once they saw the probable stroke they gave me a cerebral angiogram, an x-ray with dye that highlights the blood vessels in the brain. It revealed "occlusion of the basilar artery with no significant flow to the superior cerebellar arteries." An occlusion is the blockage of an artery and those are important brain arteries. Then doctors gave me a magnetic resonance imaging (MRI) scan and found "large bilateral infarcts in the pons and midbrain," clots blocking some arteries and depriving part of my brain of oxygen. That is the textbook definition of a stroke. At nineteen, I had had a stroke and was in a coma.

7
Friends

Merriam-Webster defines a friend as "a person who you like and enjoy being with: a person who helps or supports someone."[3] They should add, the person you party with.

I had plenty of friends and hung out with lots of people. My best friends were Breanna (Bre), Savanna (Savi), and Trav. Dee and Laci and I mostly hung out to party.

Bre and I have been friends since elementary school. We drifted apart, found each other again, and were inseparable during our junior year of high school. For our senior trip we drove down to Daytona Beach, Florida. My uncle let us use his beach condo for a week. For the first few days Bre and I had the room to ourselves, then her boyfriend and two of his friends joined us. Our beer wall was huge!

Bre was the "'yin to my yang," as ridiculous as that sounds. If I felt like being my introvert self, she could drag me out of the house and spur my extrovert personality. It was always Bre who helped me calm my perfectionist and control freak tendencies. One time during a panic attack I began to hyperventilate. She stood in front of me, telling me to match my breathing to hers. Although five other people were rubbing my shoulders and patting my back, watching Bre breathe was the only thing that calmed me.

This story will make you laugh, but the strict schedule person in me still gets upset by it. Sometimes I would give Bre a ride to school. The night before, I made sure to call her and say, "I'll be at your house around 8:05.

Please be ready." I arrived promptly, and what happened every friggin' time? She would still be in the house, sleeping...*sleeping!* Not running around getting ready, but still curled up under the covers in a full-on, deep sleep! Needless to say, I learned my lesson quickly and arrived earlier.

Savi takes the honors as my next-longest friend. We met the first day of sixth grade. Our sophomore year of high school we took the forty-five-minute drive to Dad's medical office to get our belly buttons pierced! One of the other doctors in the office had experience piercing body parts—she had pierced her own belly button, so we were her next trial.

Savi and I both have adoptive dads, so that attached us hip to hip all through middle school and most of high school. We could and still do, occasionally, turn to each other with biological father and stepdad frustrations. Sometimes it's hard to deal with the fact that your biological father chooses not to be a part of your life.

One time a friend asked me how to tell her daughter that her dad doesn't want her at all in his life. Straightaway I said, "Don't tell her that." Somebody telling you your dad doesn't want you and knowing it yourself in your heart are two different things entirely.

I partied with all my friends, but the first time I got drunk was with Savi. It was the night before Mother's Day, and I had recently turned fifteen. Savi came over to my house to bake and decorate cakes for our moms. Mine was on call and had to go in to work a few hours.

The older, intelligent me would say, "It's only a couple of hours. Finish the cake," but the teenaged me said, "Mom's gone—let's drink!" I ran to retrieve a fifth of tequila from its hiding place in my room. A few weeks earlier we had asked a friend over twenty-one to buy it for us. I poured the liquor. Savi had to drive home later, so she was smart enough not to drink.

We followed our recipes and made the cakes; mine just looked a little ruff compared to Savi's. After about an hour of me drinking half the bottle, Savi realized, "Oh shit! You're drunk and your mom is coming home soon!" Neither of us was an experienced drinker, so she called our friend Matt and prayed he knew what to do.

"She has to sober up," he said. "Make her throw up."

Oh how I wish Savi had given me something gross to drink and I had proceeded to hurl.

But that's not what truly happened...

Savi decided, for some reason, to put me in the passenger seat of her car. She handed me a bucket. Then she drove, intermittently slamming on the brakes, pitching me violently forward. Luckily, our little excursion occurred at night, but my neighbors probably thought, *What the hell?*

When Savi's plan failed (I didn't throw up), we went back to my house. Just as we got inside, we looked out the window of the front door and saw Mom's car pulling in the driveway. I started to laugh hysterically as Savi began to push me up the stairs to my room. She threw me in my bed and tried to hold me down as I tried to sit up. We heard Mom come in and we started whisper-yelling at each other.

"Quit it! I can act sober."

"No you can't! Shut up and lay here. I have to go home."

Our living room had an open ceiling with a balcony right outside my bedroom door. Mom yelled up to my room, "Girls, I'm back!"

Savi left me in bed and walked to the door. "Hi, Karen. I think I'm going to head home now. Jess isn't feeling good."

I jumped out of bed, ran past Savi, and screamed, "'Hi, Mom! I'm so glad you are back!" Whoops—busted. Actually, the busting came hours later when she heard me throwing my guts up.

Shortly after that cluster, Savi and I experienced another cluster of her teaching me to drive stick shift.

My dad was adamant: "If you get stuck somewhere you have to know how to drive any kind of car in any kind of weather." He tried to teach me, but our similar personalities just made us scream and argue the whole time: "Dammit, Sissy, I said let the clutch out slow!"

"Would you shut the hell up, Dad! I am trying to do that!"

Late one night we went to practice in the parking lot of Savi's church. Thankfully, I learned quickly. I guess the years spent changing gears with my foot on our four-wheeler helped.

It's a coin toss between Trav and Laci regarding who comes next for the longest friendship. All of us met in middle school, but I don't remember who came first. It's funny to see old pictures of us from back then. We look so young and innocent.

Laci and I had several classes in common, but Trav and I only had one semester of Spanish together. In that class he earned the nickname *Trabajar* (Spanish for "to work").

One day the teacher asked Trav to fix something on the TV as she walked into the other room. He pushed the wrong button and the TV blared white noise. She ran back into the room with her hands above her head, screaming, "¡*Trabajar!* ¡*Ay Dios mío!*" (Oh, my God!). Hilarious! That day was forever known as "The day *Trabajar* messed up *Señora Consuelos'* TV."

Trav and I hung out every day after school watching TV and movies. A lot of nights he came to our house for dinner or I went out to eat with his family—they didn't cook often. One dinner we teased his aunt and sister. I stuck out my stomach and Trav rubbed it while we both said, "We have some news!"

For the longest time I couldn't watch *A League of their Own* without crying, remembering us quoting every line. Remember the girl on *Real World: Hawaii* who would scream "Spooooon me!" to her boyfriend? Trav would lie on the couch and scream at me just like that girl. We hung out every day and went to Prom and Winter Formal together. Helping to decorate our high school for events like Prom and Spirit Week was always fun.

Trav was more vocal about his feelings for me than I was about mine for him. He told Mom and Bre that he loved me, but I took a passive-aggressive approach to avoid talking about our relationship. I did, however, scoff and have temper tantrums if he dated other girls.

My friend Laci happens to be tremendously smart. In high school I remember feeling miffed that she got a higher grade on a paper than me. I read an article in *Psychology Today* that said one common corollary with being smart is experimentation with drugs,[4] so maybe it makes sense that Laci took my pot smoking virginity.

Savi joined Laci and me by our pool late that night. Although Savi and I had tried to smoke pot once before, we didn't do it right because we felt nothing. You know how you're supposed to take a puff and hold it in? We didn't do that. Once Laci schooled us, the stereotypical scene occurred: puff...cough cough..."You gotta try this shit."

After we finished smoking, we grabbed some snacks from the kitchen for our munchies and snuck back to my room. We tried to giggle quietly and creep up the stairs (my parents' bedroom happened to be underneath the stairs). Once we got to my room we could finally laugh out loud and eat. Sitting cross-legged on the floor I rocked back and forth. After almost ten minutes (it might have been five to twenty minutes—who knows?) of me rocking, Laci noticed and said, "What is wrong with you? Quit it!" I didn't even notice I had been doing it—hahaha.

Dee rounds up the group of my friends. We met in high school but could talk to each other in complete gibberish. She started the language years before, but we all learned. Instead of pointing to something and saying, "Get that over there," we would point to it and say "Abuuuhh." To say "No," you would stick your index finger in the air, move it side to side, and say "Eh huh." Every time you drank (anything from milk to vodka) you would shrug your shoulders and say in a high-pitched voice, "Drinkle drinkle." Those made up the core phrases.

That sums up my friends. We experienced crazy times together, we got in trouble together, but we were always there for each other. Bre went with me to the psychologist to talk about my bulimia, and I left work to take her to the hospital when she had bad stomach cramps.

Savi and I consoled each other about friends and grandparents who passed away. Trav and I spent graduation morning taking flowers to each other's grandparent's graves. Dee drove thirty minutes to come get me because Dad and I had been fighting, and I went to her dance competitions and games. Laci and I really only partied together but she stepped up the most, as you'll read later. We took care of one another. None of us happened to be the best influence on anyone else, but we were kids.

Whereas the teenaged me thought of friends as people to party with, now I like the *Urban Dictionary's* definition of a friend: "someone who forgives you no matter what you do…someone who tries to help you even when they don't know how. A friend is someone who tells you if you're being stupid, but who doesn't make you feel stupid."[5]

8
Coma

With me hovering so close to death, my family and friends didn't know what to do or think or where to turn. Mom needed some alone time with God. She walked down the hall to a call room that the hospital gave Dad and her to use during my hospital stay. Closing and locking the door, she got down on her knees and prayed.

Mom begged God for my life. If He let her keep me, she told him, together we would make something beautiful out of this. Somehow, she knew that at that moment she could not remain a fair weather Christian. She decided to believe that God did, in fact, love us and had a good plan for our lives. That was the most important decision of our journey. From then on she decided to hang on to her Bible with both hands, not listening to people but to God.

Me, I was listening, off and on, to everyone and everything around me. I was in a coma (aka a somnolent and unresponsive state), which most people assume is like a deep sleep. According to the Mayo Clinic, signs and symptoms of a coma commonly include:

- "Closed eyes
- Depressed brainstem reflexes, such as pupils v not responding to light
- No responses of limbs, except for reflex movements
- No response to painful stimuli, except for reflex movements
- Irregular breathing"[6]

I wish my family had taken pictures of me in the hospital. I don't know what I looked like with all those tubes. They probably don't want to remember, but it would be interesting for me to see.

Vague images, sensations, and tiny snippets of conversations from my time in the Neurological ICU swirl in my memory. Like ice chips. I remember my nurse placing ice chips underneath my arms. Later I learned this was an attempt to lower my body temperature, because it got (and still gets) wacky sometimes. My stroke occurred near the hypothalamus, which regulates body temperature. One time I even remember somebody turning me in my bed to prevent bedsores. Not realizing I could hear her, she commented snarkily on my "Lucky" tattoo: "Well, she's not so lucky anymore."

During my coma I experienced several odd dreams. I dreamt of being caught in a rainy, dreary, abandoned city with my childhood friends Lisa and Maddie. Another occurred back in the 1800s with my brother and cousin. They shot somebody and threw the gun in a pond. In still another I was swimming in a lake and trying not to drown. In the most bizarre dream, I was walking along a river in Mexico with Jennifer Lopez. The people in the dreams probably had to do with the people around me at the time, except Jennifer Lopez—she must have been on TV.

Later I made the connection that all the dreams contained water, so I checked the internet on how to interpret dreams. Apparently, water dreams deal with not being able to express your emotions. Uh, no shit, Sherlock—I was in a coma!

I even experienced some out-of-body experiences. Once while I floated above my body I looked down at my friend crying over me. Not realizing it was me, I thought, *Why is Jackie crying over that girl?* Eventually, I told family and friends about conversations I heard and things I saw while in my coma. They were shocked I remembered something as little as Savi's outfit one day. You will laugh at this story: One day my "bed buddy," Brenson, visited. While talking to Granny and my body, he told her, "We used to four-wheel together." "Four-wheel" was our code word for sex. To which my soul or whatever said, *Don't you dare tell my Granny what that means!*

I know—I didn't believe in near-death experiences (NDEs) either until I experienced one. The International Association for Near Death Studies (IANDS) reports these common characteristics of NDEs:

1. Strong emotions
2. An out-of-body experience (OBE)
3. Moving through blackness, sometimes to a bright light
4. Fast-paced thinking
5. Reaching a spiritual realm

6. Meeting loved ones who have died
7. A life review
8. Sudden realizations about the nature of life
9. A decision to return to consciousness[7]

The first four events were part of my NDE. It ended when I heard a voice (like the blind kid on *Dumb and Dumber* talking to the bird) saying, "Pretty girl! Wake up, pretty girl."

Once I fell into the "deep sleep," Mom kept a daily journal; later it helped jog my memory when I was writing this book. She wrote that I cried a good deal in the weeks I spent asleep but never opened my eyes. A pea-sized blood clot in the reticular formation network in my brain stem prevented blood from flowing and simultaneously affected my awake/sleep schedule;[8] hence the weeks of my deep sleep. Unfortunately, the clot was inoperable. Doctors could only push blood thinners and wait. Everyone prepared for the worst—that I might never wake up, or if I did it would almost certainly be with irreversible brain damage.

Everyone had an opinion about the best course of action if the worst occurred.

Mom's response to the pessimistic doctors was, "Well, if she doesn't wake up, I will just take care of her forever."

Aunt Kristen took the opposite approach and told the doctors, "God has a lot of questions to answer about this!"

I didn't know this story until recently, but the neurologist told Granny, "Your daughter knows what she needs to do," implying Mom should pull the plug on me.

When I entered the coma, no one knew the outcome. My parents and Blake sat at my bedside holding my hands and talking to me, Dad saying how much he loved me and, "You're the smartest and best kid any parent could ever ask for." Blake looked up and said, "What about me?" Hahaha!

It still kills me to think how close my family and friends came to losing me. My parents almost lost a daughter, my brother almost lost a sister, my friends almost lost a friend. *Almost.*

On April 6th, after floating in the coma for two weeks and five days, I opened my eyes, looked around, and tried to see where I was. Not knowing what had happened to me, I had the following conversation with myself in my head:

Where am I? Argh! Dammit, I can't see shit! I gotta find my contacts or glasses. I probably just fell asleep somewhere strange. *That is* so *responsible, Jessica. Okay, time to get up. You're acting stupid. Get up! Okay, this isn't funny. What the hell is going on? OMG, why can't I get up or talk?*

I just lay there and cried my eyes out. To give you a funny visual of the difficult situation, it felt like that scene in the movie A *Christmas Story* where the little brother, stuffed into his snowsuit, falls and gets stuck in the snow.

When I woke I only remember Dad. Overcome with excitement, he kept getting in my face yelling, "Great! You're awake! Cry! Show me you can cry!"

Because it was all I could do, I cried. I know he felt excited I woke up, but the more he said it the more frustrated I became. Crying was my only option and I hated it. Some other family members were in the room, but he is the only person I vividly remember.

After I opened my eyes, they moved me from the Neuro ICU to the Intensive Care Unit (ICU), where I could finally have visitors other than family. My mom called a few of my friends. In minutes, just about my entire graduating class from high school and several of my teachers were in the hall to see me. That shows you how small my childhood town is—you tell one person something and suddenly *everybody* knows. The nurses were shocked by the crowd. My mom and Granny made people come in in twos.

Along with the journal Mom wrote herself, she also kept a notebook beside my bed for my friends to write in. Their notes varied from "I am praying for you" to "You can pull through this" *to my neighbor Wyatt writing, "Get up you know you want a cigarette." One day while penning a message, Trav stopped and said to Mom, "Can I write, 'You better not fudgen' die'?"*

    Basically, the hospital royally fudged up my case. First, the radiologist who reviewed my second CT read it wrong (even though he asked for help to interpret it correctly). Second, during the early stages of my stroke the ER doctors neglected to give me a medicine called tissue plasminogen activator (tPA) that might have dissolved the clot. Third, the MRI they gave me on March 22 was five long days after my stroke and too late to have been any use in preventing adverse effects. Overall, it took much too long to diagnose me.

    My family and I started to sue but didn't follow through. Our lawyer was a divorce lawyer with no experience in medical law, and once we moved up north it just wasn't a top priority anymore. Now it's past the statute of limitations. "But…it could have helped; you all *could* have tried harder," some people say. Because we didn't finish the lawsuit, I didn't sign a gag clause; thus I am able to discuss how much the hospital and doctors screwed up and how after my stroke they conveniently developed a stroke center in their ER.

    Most of my family remains much more upset than I am regarding the predicaments that occurred. They would rather blame, whereas I think that this was supposed to happen. It is my belief that God lets bad things happen sometimes for a greater reason. Mistakes don't just happen for shits and giggles—there's a reason why. We could have showcased and blamed everyone involved for their negligence, and they might have made things worse for me. But they didn't cause my stroke, and it's because of them I'm alive.

9
Big

High school zoomed by in a blur of parties, drunken nights, and time spent with family and friends that I'll never forget. I definitely needed a bit of maturing, and taking on a job right before my senior year of high school helped a lot in that department. One of my first positions was grill cook at a restaurant called Steak 'n Shake. After I worked the grill and served in other parts of the kitchen, the general manager asked me to take some classes and become a production manager. Basically, I was a real manager. I closed or opened the restaurant, helped hire people, handled money, and waited tables if needed. It was a lot of responsibility for an eighteen-year-old, but I welcomed it.

Luckily, my high school let you graduate early if you were able to complete all your credits. All through middle and most of high school I had been called "the rich girl" or "the doctor's daughter." When you come from a family full of doctors and people in the medical field, you do get medical questions answered quickly, haha, but being singled out every day for it becomes annoying and rather embarrassing. It sounds ridiculous that a childish taunt motivated me to graduate early, but it did. That and the regular old high school attitude of being eager to be finished with school made me work my ass off to earn all my credits. Even though I graduated in December of 2002, I still went to prom and our big graduation in May 2003.

I breezed through my senior year, taking two classes in the morning then leaving to do my third class, Senior Project. I researched culinary schools around the country and visited local restaurants to shadow and interview the chefs. An aspiring chef's dream!

After graduating a semester early, I worked every day at Steak 'n Shake to save money for college. Bre, along with my parents, convinced me to stay in-state and get my bachelor's degree before going to culinary school. My parents' argument was, "You can be a chef, but be an educated chef" (get your nutrition degree first). Thinking back, I realize they probably worked together and tricked me to change my mind. It ended up being a good decision, though. My dad and I had been fighting a lot, so I was excited to go to school with Bre one-and-a-half hours away.

Nearly a month before school started, we had an orientation weekend where you meet some classmates (scope out the hotties, haha) and get to know the layout of the campus. Bre and I felt excited about the visit! We drove around the campus and nearby town, proud of becoming adults moving away from home and into the dorm. A few months before our trip I bought a video camera; it's funny to see Bre and me point out the town's numerous places for us to work while in school.

Move-in day for East Tennessee State University that August was blazing hot. Trav and Mom moved me into the dorm. Thankfully (sarcastically said), the elevator in the dorm broke, so we lugged all my shit up five floors! Trav kept walking behind me whispering, "Let me not walk beside you and cock block for you." I managed to hold back my tears hugging Mom and Trav bye, but later that night driving around with Bre, I lost it.

My sobs alternated with gasps of air: "I have (gasp) to go (gasp) home. Blake (gasp) needs me. We don't (gasp) know anybody."

Bre (yin to my yang) looked me in the eye, saying, "Jess, you're fine. Quit crying." Fast forward two hours, as we began meeting dormmates—I was smiling again. The one good thing about smoking is that it is a social habit. You sit outside and meet people.

My course load that semester included Sociology, English, Computer, Nutrition, and Weight Management (gym). Each class took place in a different building, so I walked around campus a lot every day. Since my classes weren't grueling, I had time for a rich social life.

Luckily our dorm was co-ed, so the guys and girls on our floor and all over the building became fast friends. I still talk to some of the girls. Most of the guys were just friends, haha! (I made out with several guys before dating Samuel, then didn't after).

Samuel and I met right after college started. He roomed with Bre's boyfriend, Charlie, in an apartment ten minutes from my house. Dee, Bre, and I went there to see it (and honestly, to drink.) The minute we met, I did the girly smile with the head tilt: "Hi I'm Jessica!" We instantly became a thing.

I can't remember precisely when I started birth control. I was about sixteen, sexually active, and in no position to be anyone's mom. Had the stroke not happened, I am certain I would have ended up a young mother like several of my friends. The jury is still out on whether I'd have been a good one. Even on birth control, I had a pregnancy scare in college. Shortly after meeting Samuel, I switched birth control methods. We broke up, I was late, and I freaked. Then, to boot, my college roommate was feeling my stomach and felt a knot in my uterus. Looking back now, I'm glad something took me off that path, but leave it up to God to make it so drastic.

The first weekend after school started, some students drove by our dorm and said, "Hey y'all, there's a party at OML (a chapter of Alpha Phi Alpha Fraternity) house!" That one invitation led to my friends and me going there about three days a week. A lot of people at school, including me, went home every weekend, so the big party night was Thursdays. If OML wasn't hosting a party, we would go to a bar with the brothers.

One night after starting to date Samuel, I went to OML and got really drunk—on hard liquor instead of my usual beer. Wasted, I went outside to the garage by myself and just lay on the cold concrete floor. I fell asleep for a few minutes—or almost dozed off (I don't remember).

Samuel got soooo mad at me. "Dammit, Jessica! They could have done something to you!"

I scoffed. "No they wouldn't. They are like brothers!" We had several fights about me getting drunk with the OML brothers.

It was while in college that I decided to switch from birth control pills to the ring. My friend from across the hall in my dorm suggested this new ring-shaped birth control you only had to change every three weeks instead of remembering to take a pill every day. I didn't always remember to take my birth control pills and taking them at the exact same time every day was impossible. This new ring sounded like it could make me much more accountable—and in much less danger of getting pregnant.

The nurse at the college medical center just gave it to me. Seriously, no questions, no explanations, just a quick Pap smear and, "Here you go, Sweetie." The package did come with that skinny folded paper with the small print, but please tell me what eighteen-year-old reads that *whole* thing. Or whether I would have understood any of the legalese even if I had? Who would have thought that such a simple process, such an offhanded decision, would cause my life to spin so out of control? Trust me, I didn't.

10
School's Out

College seemed to bring another welcome period of maturation, settling me down (a little). Yet at the same time college allowed me to escape responsibilities and remain a teenager—drink a lot, act stupid, and make out with lots of guys (surprisingly, I didn't sleep around during college, haha). The maturing was really only doing my own laundry and cooking, along with acting as "the Mom" to my friends when they got drunk or sick. One night I stumbled back to the dorm with Bre, both of us sloshed. "Well, you can't be the Mom tonight," she said.

For the first few weeks of school Bre and I lived together, but I moved out to save our friendship. We fought every day, and our opposite personalities almost killed each other. She didn't mind the room messy, but I wanted it clean and organized. I preferred to go to bed early and to be in class early, but she liked to stay up late and roll in late to class. We both drank; I just thought it was better to get sloshed on the weekend.

Along with calling home every day, I went home most weekends to check on and hang out with my family, friends, and Samuel. The guys at the frat we frequented always teased me about going home to Mommy, but they didn't know what my home life truly entailed. School was my reprieve. Going home every weekend pretty much tore me apart.

Blake was active in baseball and football and didn't drive yet, so I was his chauffeur to games and tournaments and the face of our family cheering him on. And although he was old enough to babysit himself, being six years older I still felt very maternal toward him, making sure he kept up with his schoolwork and stayed out of trouble. He used to tell Mom, "Sissy's like my other Mommy."

Then there was Dad. He had started using drugs when I was in high school. As his drug use accelerated, his medical practice declined, and the daily household and financial responsibilities fell onto Mom. Every weekend I saw her running around like crazy, juggling a fulltime job, housework, errands, doing things with Blake... She never complained, but I saw the toll it took on her. What she couldn't handle, I volunteered to do. That probably planted my maternal seed with Blake. Truthfully, I felt like the character Fiona from the TV show *Shameless,* trying to keep my family together while whoring around trying to find a man better than Dad.

It's embarrassing how much Dad and I fought. And it hurts to remember how fun and loving we used to be and how everything changed.

Growing up, I embraced being a total Daddy's Girl, permanently attached to his hip. Strangers in the grocery store would say to us, "You can tell who her daddy is!" During his medical residency he worked many long hours at a time. I begged him, "Quit and work at McDonald's so I can get free Happy Meals."

As a preschooler I lived for the days Dad drove me to school. My mom always took me early, but he let me sleep in. We shared a late breakfast at the diner down the street and came strolling into school around noon. He was probably tired from working late in the ER, but it made for good memories.

In elementary school we stayed close. Dad would pick me up from middle school in his fancy car and show it off for my classmates. As soon as we got home I would yell, "Mom! Dad brought the Viper and embarrassed me again!"

His drug use continued through college. Our connection dissolved and I boiled with anger towards him. We argued about everything, getting into horrendous screaming matches about anything from the hairdryer to me missing work, mostly because we share the same take-no-BS personality. The more we argued, the more promiscuous I became.

The maternal me loved taking care of Blake, but the teenaged me went berserk being trapped at home—and blamed Dad. We both have bad tempers, and my crazy moods—ranging from normal to angry to depressed—made things worse. Hormonal birth control can cause mood swings, and I believe my birth control exacerbated this situation.

Have I mentioned that I am a perfectionist? When my family started going to crap, I took it hard, putting everything on my shoulders. Alcohol became a good friend. In high school I drank for fun, but in college I drank to drown feelings of anger and misery. I drank excessively every chance I could. Instead of going to the library to study, I spent most weekdays drinking at the frats and showing the brothers my cleavage. I drank much more than the average college partier, even more than the average college binge drinker. Samuel was twenty-one so I stayed at his apartment and drank all weekend. Bre and Mom each noticed and questioned me. When I wasn't drinking I was arguing with Dad.

One time I was watching Oprah (when it aired every day), and an alcoholic woman said how many beers she drank each day. I thought, "Holy crap! I drank twice that."

While college life and responsibilities at home consumed me and I kept consuming alcohol, I never stopped to think about what I truly wanted out of school or life. My parents had picked my major for me and the study of nutrition wasn't my passion (I practiced bulimia, remember? I wasn't exactly living a nutritious lifestyle). I needed time to sit and think about what the heck I wanted to major in. That was a big factor in my decision to leave the university. But my family situation put me over the top and became my excuse to leave school. The break would give me much needed time to reevaluate what I truly wanted out of life.

It was an easy decision, but one of the smartest stupid ones I've ever made. I know, total oxymoron—but let me explain. At first glance, dropping out of school after just one semester seems unwise and irresponsible; I love school and could have given it a better shot. Moreover, my family didn't appreciate my decision and were livid with me for a few months. But let's face it—had I stayed, my roommate, Andi, would most likely have found me dead in our dorm room from the stroke. So in that sense, it was one of the best decisions I could have made. You're welcome, Andi.

11

Up

Moving home from college with my tail between my legs dashed all my big plans. I guess it's true what John Lennon said about life happening while you're making other plans. I was pretty pissed for a while.

Weirdly enough, once I came home things started to fall into place and work out perfectly. Home still felt miserable (Dad and I would just as soon scream insults as say hello), but everything else took an upswing. I trained for a new job, Trav and I planned to get an apartment together, and one of my childhood friends, Lisa, asked me to be one of her bridesmaids!

The job was a step up from my gig at good ol' Steak 'n Shake at seventeen. I called it semi-upscale because to wait tables I had to wear black pants, a white button-up shirt and a long men's tie. It was just another job, but I was excited about it, and it was perfect for me at the moment.

Then on to apartment hunting. Once I moved back home, Trav and I spent every single day together, so becoming roommates seemed like a natural decision. We knew this lady who managed apartments, and they just so happened to be located in the part of town we liked!

We looked at three apartments, but each had some major flaw. Discouraged and about to give up, we pulled up to one last building and saw the unkempt outside.

Right away, Trav said, "No, it's ugly."

I retorted, "Well, don't judge a book by its cover. Let's just look."

It fit us to a T—first floor, a big bedroom for each of us, a deck off the living room for parties. The only detail that bothered me was an oddly-placed window near the floor of the kitchen. Weird, right? I sometimes babysat our friend Susie's son and that window worried me. If he crawled and fell out that window, I would surely get the Worst Babysitter of the Year award. We decided we could block the window when Pat came over. It was perfect.

Next on the agenda: Lisa's wedding! My twin friends, Lisa and Maddie, and I had remained friends since elementary school and made a pact as kids to be in one another's weddings. We picked Lisa's wedding gown, and after several tries we picked our bridesmaids' dresses. Everything was set. The perfectionist was finally getting her perfect life.

But I never got to wear that pink spaghetti-strap bridesmaid dress.

12
The Perfect Storm

Stroke respects no age limits. Even an infant can suffer one. But in children, strokes usually result from trauma such as a neck injury or congenital conditions such as hemophilia, sickle cell disease, or an abnormal heart valve. The age group most at risk for stroke is those over fifty-five. Otherwise-healthy nineteen-year-olds like me do not usually show up in the ER with stroke symptoms. So even when an MRI showed "large bilateral infarcts" (blood clots) in my brain, the doctors didn't immediately understand why. My uncle, an anesthesiologist, and his friend, a gynecologist, finally figured it out.

My uncle and his friend realized that several women in my family have suffered multiple miscarriages, which sometimes occur because of a blood clotting disorder. My uncle told my doctor, who sent my blood to another hospital to get checked, and lo and behold! I have a blood disorder called Prothrombin 20210 that causes clots to form.

Out of 1000 individuals with Prothrombin 20210, only two or three will develop a blood clot.[9] However, the risk increases if you smoke or take birth control as I did. If I had done one or the other—smoking, but no birth control or birth control, but no smoking—I would have had a small chance of developing a blood clot. However, the combination made me a ticking time bomb.

That explains the blood clot, but why the stroke? A tiny hole in my heart was the culprit. A patent foramen ovale (PFO) is a hole in the heart that didn't close the way it should have after birth. All through fetal development, a small flap-like opening—the foramen ovale—is normally present in the wall between the right and left upper chambers of the heart. It usually closes in infancy. When the foramen ovale doesn't close, it's called a patent foramen ovale. Dr. Patrick O'Gara, professor of medicine at Harvard Medical School and executive director of the Shapiro Cardiovascular Center, explains that "PFOs don't actually cause strokes, but they provide a portal through which a thrombus (blood clot) might pass from the right to the left side of the circulation."[10] The clot can travel to the brain, causing a stroke or transient ischemic attack (TIA). If it stays in the heart or goes to the lungs, causing a pulmonary embolism, it can cause irregular heartbeat, shortness of breath, spitting up blood, or death.[11]

Truth be told, my uncle's friend hit the ceiling that my doctor didn't figure out sooner instead of days later (three, to be exact) that I had had a stroke—and why. I have seen multiple doctors since my stroke, and they have confirmed that the combination of birth control, smoking, and my blood disorder created the clot, and my PFO became the tunnel to my brain.

Somebody anonymously emailed me and questioned the truth of what caused my stroke, so let me repeat: My doctors, including my hematologist, affirmed that the combination of birth control, smoking, and my blood disorder created the clot, and my PFO became the tunnel to my brain. That's why at nineteen, I had a stroke.

13
Accepted

Only two percent of people survive brain stem strokes.[12] The brain stem is the base of the brain that connects to the spinal cord. It controls basic body functions such as consciousness, breathing, heart rate, blood pressure, breathing, swallowing, and wakefulness.[13] My stroke was located in the brain stem.

Hospital ER staff uses the Glasgow Coma Scale (GCS) to rate your alertness as you physically deteriorate. When you're alert and normal your score is 15, and 3-8 when comatose. According to Dad, my GCS started at 14 and was eventually recorded as a 3 when I was comatose. The Mayo Clinic defines coma as a "state of prolonged unconsciousness" in which a person does not respond normally to sensory stimuli and has depressed brainstem reflexes.[14]

Once I was in a coma I transitioned from the hospital to its rehabilitation facility. All those years Mom worked in that hospital, and I had no clue one of the top rehabilitation centers in the south bustled two floors above. Now that is just wrong for me not knowing.

April 17, 2004 was the big day! Big as in reflective of my progress. The center had all these entrance requirements, and they accepted me (It's weird that I'm talking about getting into rehab like getting into college, but that was my "new normal").

Mom put it this way: "If they didn't feel they could rehabilitate you, then they wouldn't have accepted you." That gave me hope in a bleak situation.

At first they didn't know where to put me. The rehab center bedrooms were divided by age. Most of the older people had had strokes while the young people suffered from spinal cord injuries and brain damage. But a nineteen-year-old with a stroke...ummm?? Ultimately, I was housed with the younger folks, but my physical therapy floated between the stroke and spinal cord injury floors.

My memory of my transition from the hospital to rehab remains foggy, but I do remember one funny story. The staff told my family I needed workout clothes and shoes. Although I owned suitable clothes, my shoes didn't fit well anymore, so Granny volunteered to go shopping for me. She didn't know what shoes I would like, so she asked my friend Dee, who was visiting at the time. Dee told my grandmother to get me some white high tops with some scrunch socks. So not in style in 2004!

I was on morphine, my neck and jaw clenched up, so I looked out of it but wasn't. In my head I screamed, *Granny, she's joking! Dammit Dee—tell her you're joking! Don't get me those ugly ass shoes!*

That story sounds hilarious to me now, but I fumed at the time. A couple years ago, Dee told me she used the shoes as a joke, hoping to get me to talk.

To help me breathe during my coma and the first day or two of rehab, I had a tracheotomy. This is surgery in which an incision is made through the neck into the trachea. A tube is connected and breathing occurs through it, rather than through the nose and mouth.[15] My family prayed every day for me to get strong enough to do anything by myself: breathe, swallow—anything. On April 18th God answered that prayer. I don't recollect having the trach, but I do remember getting it out!

Granny stayed in my hospital room with me one night, and when she woke she saw my trach hanging half out. She screamed for the nurses, and they called my doctor to fix it. He got the emergency call from home and came running into my room in shorts and a t-shirt.

Seeing me *not* gasping for air he said, "Well, Jessica, looks like you are breathing fine without this," and yanked it out! Granny and I remember me jumping nearly a foot off the bed! She called Mom and said, "You got your miracle. Jess can breathe on her own."

My close friends responded differently to my stroke: Trav came every day initially, Dee and Laci came often, Savi and Bre remained sporadic, but Lisa came every day for several years. Bre regretted backing off at first and gave me a best friends locket that we each wore.

When Lisa visited and saw the locket, she took it off me and said to Mom and Granny, "Bre barely comes—that's not a best friend!"

So the joke between Mom and Granny was, whichever friend they saw walking down the hospital hall, they would put on or take off the locket. Thankfully, we have all matured since "locket gate."

A few years ago Mom and I stumbled upon this TV show on the top 100 songs of the 2000s. Around thirty of them triggered memories from the hospital for me. I remember hearing "Yeah" by

Usher on the TV in the ICU. Every morning when they got me up for rehab the TV always played "The Reason" by Hoobastank. My rehab nurse always joked with me when she turned me in bed, singing, "Which way do you want to turn? To the window, to the wall!" like the song "Get Low" by Lil Jon.

    Have you ever looked at something and expected to see something else, and it literally makes you jump? That's how it was the first time I looked in the mirror after my stroke. A bit dramatic maybe, but in truth it was traumatic for me. My occupational therapist (OT), Loni, wanted me to try to wash my hands in the bathroom. She didn't think about there being a mirror in that particular bathroom (in the hospital not every sink had a mirror), or that I hadn't looked in the mirror yet.

    The minute we entered the bathroom and I saw my reflection, I started to scream and cry. I looked nothing like I had looked for nineteen years before. It appeared as if the left side of my face was dead and the right was waking up from an all-night bender. Even today it is difficult for me to even glance in the mirror. People tell me that my face is symmetrical, but I disagree. Old pictures of me are displayed all over my room, and my face doesn't look balanced the way it used to. I'll look in the mirror now, but quickly, and not every day. You probably think I'm vain, but *oh well!*

For about a year after my stroke, I couldn't eat food by mouth, so I received nourishment through a tube in my stomach called a percutaneous endoscopic gastrostomy (PEG) tube. My caregivers squirted water into my PEG tube and then used a machine to slowly push in TwoCal, a high-calorie liquid food. To this day I have no clue what the stuff tastes like, because they squeezed it directly into my stomach. I lost around twenty pounds in the hospital, so that felt great! (I have got to make some silver lining out of this whole fiasco.) The scar from the tube in my stomach is a daily reminder of the lifesaving goop, and oddly enough, it kind of hurts when I'm starving.

They administered medicine through the PEG tube too, crushed up in water. If they squirted it in too fast I threw it up. After around a month in rehab the staff introduced me to some pureed food and thickened liquid and reduced my TwoCal, so only the speech therapist was supposed to feed me. Behind closed doors though, Mom or somebody gave me food. We were—and still are—always bending the rules, haha.

One day after my physical therapist put me over a ball for exercise, she unwittingly popped the inside part of my PEG tube and it fell out. It didn't hurt then, but *really* did later. My family—always aggressive with my rehabilitation—decided not to get it replaced. They just cut or blended my food for me and made me eat only by mouth. Although my liquids also were supposed to be thickened, they didn't fortify every drink. Again, thanks to my family's rehabilitation, I don't need my liquids thickened anymore.

Most of my food now is still cut up some. The first time Mom fed me a whole, uncut hamburger that I could bite into, she almost cried with joy. She just kept saying, "We used to feed you through a tube, and now you can eat this!"

During the months I spent in the hospital I couldn't see our dog, Harley. Though he was supposed to be Blake's dog, I fed him, took him to the groomer, and played with him. He slept with me, spent all day with me, and we felt lost without each other. That might sound ridiculous (unless you have a beloved pet), but it's true. My family told me Harley went up to my bedroom at home and curled up on my bed (*sad face*).

After I moved to the rehabilitation center my aunt Kristen took me outside for a surprise. Harley jumped on my lap and licked the tears off my face. So sweet! He needed to go to the groomer, but he was his same little Yorkie self.

On July 24th I transferred from the in-patient rehab center to an apartment-style room in the hospital—preparation for going home. Mom stayed with me, of course, but I have never understood why Dad and my brother didn't come too. Since I remained completely dependent on help at this point (you will read later about the independence I have gained), someone had to do everything for me. I needed help to feed myself, bathe, lift my head off the pillow, transfer to my wheelchair—everything.

To do my transfers you would put a gait belt under my butt, cup your knees around mine, lean me all the way forward, tuck my head under your arm, and lift my butt with the belt. It sounds and looks strenuous and uncomfortable, but it's not. Well, maybe I am just used to it, and of course I'm not the one doing the lifting. Some people (Mom) still do my transfers like that, even though I tell them it's easier now for them and me to let me stand and pivot. In the rehab, Mom would start to do a transfer, but then she would always call my nurse to do it instead.

I would think, *Dammit Mom. Buck up and do this for me.* But now it's so obvious—she felt scared. Her healthy and independent daughter was suddenly completely dependent on her for everything. That's a hard pill to swallow.

As far as rehabilitation goes, it wasn't the best idea to leave so soon, but a mixture of family situations and insurance problems made that decision for me. Even though I wouldn't be able to get the intense therapy that staying in-house would provide, we opted to commute from home to the rehab a few times a week.

One detail I learned in physical therapy: you end up in some awkward sexual positions. Sometimes you are able to laugh, and other times you can't. One time to strengthen my core my therapist suggested to his aide, "Okay, get her on all fours. I will brace the elbows so she doesn't fall, then you push up the butt." As he's bracing my elbows, the aide and I are laughing hysterically, saying, "What the hell are you doing to us? Girl-on-girl *Kama Sutra* shit!"

Another time a female PT named Allison had me doing the same exercise, but this time with two male aides. She instructed one guy to brace my elbows, then instructed the other aide, "Get behind her and push her hips back and forth and side to side." I whipped my head around and looked at her like, *Are you friggin' serious? I am going to die laughing!* She shook her head. "Never mind. I'll get **back there.**"

The day I left the hospital, July 27, 2004, I cried uncontrollably (again).

Mom got frustrated with me. "Come on, Jess. Get it together," she said.

But going home after my stroke meant that this hadn't all been a dream. I had actually suffered a stroke and had to embrace the fact that I couldn't do anything for myself. That wasn't something I was quite ready to accept. I hoped that on the way home I might magically transform back to my body before the stroke. God, what I would have given to be able to walk up the three little stairs to the front door that day. In reality, my friend's husband built a ramp for my wheelchair to get into the house. We converted our rarely used dining room at home into my hospital room. It included my feeding tube pole and a shower curtain for a door (the doorway was too wide for a real door). I guess not all dreams come true.

We all did have a bit of a party once I got home, though, even if it was against medical orders. Because of my blood disorder I have to stay on a blood thinner pill for the rest of my life, which truly isn't a big deal. It just means they draw my blood every few weeks to check it and determine my dosage of blood thinner, and I must remain mindful of what foods I eat (like limiting dark green leafy vegetables and grapefruit). Since my body wasn't used to the blood thinner yet, the staff cautioned my family not to give me alcohol. Although I can drink alcohol now (I just don't drink to cover my emotions anymore), I couldn't, then. The phlebotomist doing my final blood draw before leaving the hospital couldn't find my veins to check my blood, so a nurse was to come to my house the next day. Again she reminded us, *no* alcohol.

They still can never find my veins. Today, when someone new tries to get my blood, I say, "Good luck." They laugh at first. On the second or third attempt they say, "Wow, you weren't joking." My constantly-bruised arms and hands look like those of a drug addict.

Excited that I was finally home, Granny "kind of, sort of" broke out the blender and made margaritas and I "kind of, sort of" drank one. The next day the nurse came to draw my blood, and that night the hospital called with my results. The conversation went a little like:

"Hi, this is the lab with Jessica's results. Did she have some alcohol?"

"Uhhhh, noooo…"

"Because it shows that she consumed alcohol."

Oops—hahahahaha!

I started out the chapter barely alive, but look at me now!

14
Supernatural

Nobody expected me to wake up. The doctors, nurses, nobody. So they truly didn't know what to expect *if* I woke up. Even the doctors in my family (Dad and my uncle) felt unsure. Medically, they had grave doubts. However, knowing me as their daughter and niece, they believed I might just be strong enough to pull through.

Your brain stem regulates all the basic functions in your body (breathing, heart rate, blood pressure, swallowing) and since my stroke occurred in my brain stem, I have had to relearn a lot of things. At first I couldn't breathe or swallow on my own. The scars on my neck from my tracheotomy and on my stomach from my feeding tube are daily reminders of how far I have come.

For the duration of the coma, machines monitored my heart rate and blood pressure. Granny said that when certain people walked into the room these would go up; they would relax back down when she walked in.

After initially waking from my stroke, I pretty much just floated in and out of consciousness. My family left my TV on VH1. Sometimes my eyes would remain open and other times shut, so I guess everyone figured I wouldn't need my glasses. But FYI, I am blind as a bat; I pretty much had to just listen to the TV, although that came with its perks. Fun fact: did you know Charlie Sheen and Emilio Estevez are brothers? Who would have thought? (Individuals older than me probably scoff at my surprise!)

    My life now consists of continuing to relearn things. Walking and speaking stay at the top of my list. My coma lasted so long it weakened all of my muscles. I couldn't lift my head, could barely move my arms or legs, and needed a strap on my chest and head to sit in my wheelchair. Some muscles quickly regained strength while others have taken time. Doctors and therapists have told me that I would get back only what I recovered in the first year. I am determined to prove them wrong. I woke up, didn't I?

15
Funny Girl

I have got to admit that technology helps in a huge way with how I live my day-to-day life. Without today's technology, I would be dead. Had my stroke occurred a hundred years ago, I wouldn't be talking to you. Even if I did live, I would just be able to sit in a chair or lie in bed and do nothing. I couldn't even tell anybody to scratch my ear. Technology has made my life easier and richer!

I communicate the same as everybody else, through eye movements, head shakes, and a communication device. Except that while almost everyone else articulates sounds with their mouths (or, if they're deaf, use their hands to speak), I communicate via an electronic device called a Dynavox. It's like the speech synthesizer Stephen Hawking used.

A sensor stuck on my nose connects to a pointer on my device, letting me spell words. Thankfully, my computer has word prediction, because spelling every word character by character takes hours. I'm taking college classes again and writing papers *sucks*! (Yeah, I know every college student thinks that.) But writing via a Dynavox sucks big time even though I have become fast at "typing."

My Dynavox speaks out loud what I have written, so I can have normal conversations. If I don't have it with me, most of the people who know me know how to spell with me. It's not rocket science; you just say the alphabet and I look up for the letter.

Some people don't have the patience to spell with me though, which is infuriating. My aides tell me constantly, "For someone who doesn't talk, your sighs, grunts, and face say everything!"

One time a girl I live with was yelling and cussing at one of the aides. I just looked at her, thinking, *Why are you being such a bitch? The aide is only trying to help.*

Across the room the other aide started laughing. "Jessica Davenport," she said, "fix your face. We can see what you're thinking."

Email and text are my main forms of communication, whether it's texting my brother "Hello" or emailing a friend a dirty joke. Is it wrong that I get extremely offended when people don't email or text me back? It's like people sitting in front of me having a conversation and ignoring me (which, by the way, some people do). I'm sorry, but it's just plain rude!

As time-consuming as my Dynavox remains, I've grown rather fond of it in some ways. My biological father is Costa Rican, as I mentioned earlier, so his Latin temperament has passed down to me. It used to make me explode in anger and give me "verbal diarrhea." Truthfully, my verbal diarrhea is from Dad (stepdad) too. The man did raise me, so some of his qualities had to rub off. His fantastic negotiation skills also rubbed off and I miss them. Who wants to negotiate the price of something with a girl who uses a communication device? It takes forever when I must think about what I'm going to say and then type it letter by letter. Still, I quite adore this new way of communicating because sometimes I hit the "speak" button before thinking, and half the time you probably don't want to know this brain's first reaction. I may have lessened my verbal diarrhea, but my aides tease me for remaining a smart ass.

What I might miss more than speaking is singing. To hear songs I used to sing is heartbreaking. I remember how the notes felt in my throat. Numerous therapists have told me that because I have not talked in so long, my muscles are too weak for me to ever speak or sing again. After years of people telling me no, I have to admit I started to believe them. Then I thought, *For the past fourteen years, you have been proving people wrong. Why stop now?* Currently I practice saying my name and one-syllable words.

And then there are my spiffy wheelchairs. I have two—one manual and the other a power chair. Of course, I would rather have the use of my legs for walking, but the wheelchairs work quite nicely for now. You'd be amazed at all the adaptive equipment available for those with disabilities. Unfortunately, most of it is quite expensive, so I can't order everything.

My dream item would be a car with modifications that would let me drive. Video chat is the beneficial technology I appreciate most. I video chat with Mom, Dad, extended family, friends, and my brother constantly—anything from a quick "hello" to opening presents Christmas morning. They talk and I text my answers. Recently though, when my brother or somebody says, "Bye, love you," I've started saying, "Love you." With me, not my Dynavox, actually *speaking* the words. Though I may remain behind in a lot of ways, the way I see it, I'm right where I'm supposed to be. My life has taken a slight detour, but I was probably destined for this.

Technology has changed so much since I could walk and talk in 2004! It's funny how time flies, making it feel as though everything happened so fast. I barely used to text and now everyone texts. Only one person I knew had the internet on their phone back then and now everyone has it. When I get back to my old self, I'm going to feel so lost! My last cell phone was a black and white screen flip phone and I didn't even have a regular email address. Red Box is something I've heard of but never seen up close. I could go on and on, but you get the point. Hell, until a few months ago I hadn't gone into a convenience or grocery store in years. The place where I live owns a wheelchair-accessible van, so I asked one of the drivers to take me to Wawa. Y'all, I was grinning ear to ear the whole time! When I get my dream car, I'll be hitting Wawa every day for my Columbian coffee and mango yogurt parfait.

16
17 Again

In the 2002 movie *The Hot Chick*, a popular and kind of mean girl wakes up in the body of an older, grungy criminal. Ironically, her name is the same as mine. Although it is a comedy, the scene in which she tries to explain the switch to her best friend always brings tears to my eyes.

"It's me, Jessica!" she says, jumping up and down, waving her arms, crying.

I felt like the movie Jessica after my stroke. Although I look different on the outside now, on the inside I am jumping up and down, waving my arms, screaming, "Hey! I'm here! It's still me!"

A lot of things changed after the stroke, not just how people saw me and treated me. Not a wounded puppy who needed people's pity, I was physically disabled, yet mentally the same. Yet truthfully, I didn't feel the same. I was and remain unable to speak or walk and things weren't going to get better any time soon. It was a *very* hard and confusing time. How could I face my peers without feeling insignificant and useless? My self-esteem really took a blow, and it would be a long time before I could get back a glimmer of what I used to have.

Along with the loss of some friends and some family, I lost myself. All I used to know, all that I used to be changed. It was hard for me to accept at first, and at times it still is. Losing my independence also screwed with my sense of who I was. I have always been independent. Hell, I always bragged that my parents had let me fly alone from

Tennessee to Pennsylvania to visit my grandparents since I was eight. Because I wanted my own money, I had worked since I was sixteen. So to have this body that doesn't function correctly all the time, to need someone to help me with feeding, bathing, toileting, exercising—everything—just plain sucks! I needed to get away from everyone who knew me before the stroke and find myself again.

Yet through my self-doubt and my struggle to regain my independence, my core qualities—the things that make me *me*—never changed. Because I stayed ridiculously anal, I made y'all a chart to see how I am different but the same.

Topics	Before Stroke	After Stroke
Physical strength	I was strong.	I remain oddly strong sometimes. When my aide/friend Nataja and I arm wrestled I won quickly. She was flabbergasted by my brute strength.
Mental flexibility	I demanded perfection.	Obviously, still the same. I cried multiple times in PT because I didn't think I walked/exercised well enough.
Emotional stability	I got mad or cried quickly.	Still the same. Countless times I exploded on people with anger or tears, only to apologize after.

Social development	I lit up around friends.	I remain a box full of smiles and giggles among friends.
Spiritual beliefs	I believed in God.	I believe in and trust God.
Sense of humor	I made light of uncomfortable situations.	I will leave it to you to decide whether I kept it.
Hopes and dreams	I just wanted a happy future.	I still want that, whatever it entails.
Pain threshold	I could suck up pain, if needed.	I still suck up most pain.
Anger triggers	It made me mad when people were mean to people with disabilities. (Ironic, right? Seriously, I wrote that in a book for school once.)	Now that I have disabilities, I hate when people are mean to me, whether it's not having patience or just being rude.
Worries	I worried about dying before my time.	I still worry about that but understand when it's your time, it's your time.

I thought I was different on the outside now, but it turns out some outside qualities are the same too. People tell me I laugh the same and still look just like Mom. Before the stroke I sometimes unknowingly bore a certain devilish smile. While looking through old pictures my aide and friend Nataja saw me doing that face in a picture.

"So that's where that face started!" she said.

Another time I was on video chat with a friend from high school I hadn't seen since the stroke. He told a dirty joke and I laughed and blushed.

"Yes!" he exclaimed. "You still blush for my jokes!"

Certain things from the chart, like my worries and anger triggers, changed slightly. For example, I used to worry about dying young but have learned it just means before your time and not necessarily your age. When it's your time, it's your time. Age doesn't matter when God calls you home.

Although I get angry about how people treat individuals with disabilities, I developed that trait long before my stroke. In middle school I had a class in which we tutored special ed students. It was *so* much fun! I became close with the students and teachers quickly and used to get so mad when others wouldn't take the time to truly get to know the students. Now I loathe when people see only the exterior version and don't get to truly know the real me. The outside is just one tiny facet of who I am—it's like my foot belongs in this pile while the rest of me belongs in ten other piles.

I used to flirt without realizing its effect, and I still flirt unknowingly sometimes. I would be all smiles and giggles and touchy around guy friends, then they would try to kiss me or something and we'd have that awkward moment of, "Ohh...I was joking." Remember Brenson from chapter 8? That happened with him. I was joking and then he tried to kiss me. At first I backed away and then thought, *It's just a kiss.* One time recently a former aide I hadn't seen in a while came to visit everybody. As soon as I saw him I started giggling and grabbing his hand. After five minutes of talking he said, "Jessica, girl, you are giggling at me like we're at a bar!" I immediately said I couldn't help it. So I still flirt with people unwittingly.

17
The Ugly Truth

"As life changes so will your circle."[16] These words of wisdom came to me via that great font of self-help, Pinterest. The writer must have had my circle in mind. This is hard for me to say, but it is the ugly truth of this shit storm: Everybody who knew me before the stroke treats me differently now—some better, some worse, and some don't even talk to me at all. There will be people who take offense at this, but it's the honest, "swear on a Bible" truth. I cried about it so much that it doesn't bother me anymore. Okay, I am lying. It still hurts sometimes. It's just another one of those things I have to deal with.

My relationship with Mom remains strong, but it's different since my stroke. Now she's Mom, friend, and caregiver. Sometimes I just wish we could yell at each other like normal mothers and daughters! We didn't fight much before and rarely do now, but I wish she would treat me the same as my brother. Don't call me his little sister when I'm six years older! Sure, he's twenty-seven now but I am an adult just as much as he is. If only it could stay "normal," if there even is a thing. When my stroke first happened, Mom felt frustrated and mad about me and other things. Then the first week we moved to Pennsylvania, her attitude changed and I got Mom back! The mom from before my stroke.

Now to my brother: as much as I hate what happened to me, I feel worse for what it did to him. After my stroke, nobody went to Blake's baseball games, picked him up from school, or surprised him to get him out early.

It's like everybody froze after my stroke. I got the glamorous teen years and he got the shitty ones. I had a graduation party, but did he? No. My prom and dances were a big deal, but were his? No. Just thinking about how different our teen years were makes me feel like it was my fault for all my brother went through.

My friend Nataja once asked me, "What would be the one day you would redo? Not necessarily change, just redo." It would be the day I spent with my brother for his birthday right before my stroke. You would think it would be the day of my stroke, but it's not. I can't say I much remember that day.

Post-stroke, my relationship with my brother is great, but different as well. We remain close, but at the same time there is distance that never existed before. It's the six hundred miles between us, he claims, but I noticed it even before I moved. Before and since my stroke, Blake is still the only man I can cuddle up next to and sleep like a log. With anyone else, it's "This is my side of the bed and that's yours." When we were younger, coming up to my room to watch a movie with his Sissy was a monthly treat for both of us. And as childish as this may sound, all I truly want is to be able to cuddle and take a good nap with my little brother!

My relationship with Dad is another book entirely. Long story short, he cleaned up his drug problem and found God. I can't lie and BS the truth—it has been hard for me to forgive him. We are working on our relationship, but I can't drop my shield all the way. He was an addict for many years before and after my stroke, and it's not something I can just push under the rug. Thankfully, he quit practicing medicine before it got bad. Mom and Blake have forgiven him, but they didn't go through what I have. Before my stroke I protected my brother from the truth and the arguments.

After the stroke I was the one who needed protecting, but nobody did.

Mom and Blake could just up and drive off in the car when they wanted, but I had to stay and hear, "The stroke was completely your fault because you smoked. Nobody comes around because they don't like you or even care about you." So it's going to take a long time for me to get over everything. The way I feel these days, I don't know that I ever will. Even though I want to, it's hard for me. I know now that it was the drugs making him so mean, but he still said those hurtful things. As of today, my parents are still together. They just live six hundred miles apart. I give Mom credit for sticking to her vows because I would have given up.

Every week or so since my stroke I have this reoccurring dream that somebody is trying to break into my old house. As they push the door I'm holding it and screaming for help but nobody hears me. Sometimes my brother comes and we call 911, but nobody answers. It's like my life now, in a way...

People I love really screwed me up, and I have horrible trust issues, but writing this book has been cathartic! I have been able to express out loud my frustration, anger, and hurt instead of letting it sit and stew in my stomach as it has for years. Thankfully, this has allowed me to release most of the hurt and feel inclined toward forgiving friends and family who stepped back or disappeared completely from my life. I'll admit though, friends are a lot easier to forgive than family. It's *forgiven*, but *not* forgotten.

For years I felt mad and hurt by Trav and Bre for walking out of my life. But now my over thirty-year-old self sees that it probably had to do with our age. They called less and less, then came only once a week. Their infrequent visits only occurred when Mom was home, and I would growl and think, "What the hell? You're my friend, not hers!"

When I tell my friends now about how some of my old friends quit coming around after my stroke, they always have the same reaction: "Well, I would never do that to you."

But I always think, *You aren't nineteen, and you are around people in wheelchairs every day; we weren't.* We had been around people with disabilities some, but few in wheelchairs. Bre's sister has cerebral palsy, but she's not in a wheelchair. We didn't see her as disabled, just as Bre's sister who needed help with some things, like to get back on the jet ski after she fell off.

I was strong back then. Bre's sister weighed around a hundred pounds, and I could pull her with one hand out of the water and on to our jet ski. When I worked at Steak 'n Shake I was the one girl who could lift the heavy milk bag into the milkshake stand. Even some of the guys couldn't do it. Hell yes, Girl Power! I got my power strength from Mom. We're both strong for girls. But she is getting old and losing some of her strength. Hahaha—love you, Mom!

Now the changed-for-the-better relationships...

One relationship I cherish that hasn't changed because of the stroke is the one I share with my cousin Austin. He and I have had this indescribable bond since he was little, but I didn't realize how important it was until now. The oldest grandchild on both sides of my family, I was ten when he came into the world and thirteen when he was diagnosed with autism.

Austin is nonverbal, but he uses a picture exchange communication system (PECS) to tell us what he needs. It has pictures of objects with the printed words next to them. I knew Austin could read because he would study each page of a book and then use his PECS. Years passed before everyone else could see what was plain as day to me.

Unfortunately, Austin and my other cousins lived six hundred miles away, so we only saw each other a few times a year. Still, each time it felt just as good as the time before. Sometimes he jumped up and down and yelled. To get him to stop, I would mimic him jumping and yelling. He would stop and laugh and grab my face and put it against his face. That and lightly hitting his head against yours is his way of saying, "Hi, and I love you."

When I first suffered my stroke only Austin's dad (my uncle) was able to come. Once things calmed down and I transferred to the rehabilitation center, my uncle, aunt, and cousin drove down. The second Austin saw me he jumped on my bed and grabbed my face as though nothing had changed. His parents almost had a heart attack, worried he knocked out a tube. Everybody else treated me differently, but Austin treated me the same! I didn't cry then, but I do now because it was so sweet of him.

After my stroke, when he turned eleven, Austin became able to communicate with us through spelling on a letter board. I was excited for him but thought, *No shit Sherlock, of course he knows what's going on.* He still loves to jump in my bed and bump his head against mine. He values my opinion and for that he's so cool. For that I'll always love him.

My relationships with my other cousins, and as I already told you, with my brother, remain special to me. Since for most of their lives I have lived in this post-stroke body, they don't remember much about me from before and don't compare then and now. Whether it's Olivia taking funny pictures with me or Isabella editing my English paper just because she understands how time-consuming writing is for me, they accept me for who I am now.

Truthfully, I spend much of my time with, and rely on, my aides. Often I become attached to them, and sometimes that makes people envious. In the past Mom has told me she was jealous of my relationship with an aide.

Even my hospital records mention my separation anxiety over leaving staff when being discharged.

When people just "love me for me" it's refreshing.

Fortunately, Bre and I have talked and mended our relationship, and we can forget what happened. We acknowledge our immature attitudes and how our young age affected our reactions to everything. However, the friend I still talk to the most and go places with now is Laci. She stepped up and stayed, and now we text and video chat. She came up here a few times and we even took a vacation to Washington, D.C., for the weekend (we want to plan another, but it's hard with our schedules!).

Laci explained the friend situation to me: "We left because we couldn't stand seeing how your dad and mom had been treating you."

Thinking about it made me sad and mad. It really wasn't my fault. And then I thought, *You just left?*

18

Home Is Where the Heart Is

On July 4, 2004, after months of being trapped in the hospital, Mom and my friend AJ planned "the great fireworks escape." The hospital staff informed us that we could see fireworks from the roof, but we had another idea. That evening after dark we told the rehab staff we were going to the roof, but instead snuck downstairs. From working there, Mom knew two of the night security guards, who helped AJ and Mom transfer me into AJ's car. They dropped me and I ended up with a huge bruise on my butt. *Can't I have one event that goes good?* I thought. Anyway, they got me into the car and we went to my cousin's bonfire. It was fun, if a bit awkward seeing everybody post-stroke (including a guy I kind of dated).

Languishing in the hospital day after interminable day, I wanted to go home more than a drug addict anticipating her next score, but quickly learned that home isn't always where the heart is. My family took my stroke hard at first. They acted like I died and appointed AJ to my previous spot in the family. He became Mom's movie partner and Blake's chauffer, and he made breakfast with Blake. I was just this intimate blob. And since I needed them to physically take care of me, I got the brunt of their anger and depression, and a lot of emotional abuse.

Dad's drug use had escalated since my stroke, seriously affecting our family finances. After I had been home only a few months, we sold our house and moved in with Dad's mom, Dido. That house was soooo *not* handicap accessible! A ramp was improvised to go over some dirt and stairs up to the front door. Since the stairs were steep they put a belt around my chair and hooked it to a cable and machine to tow me up the ramp. Just as you might tow a tree across your yard, they towed me—an actual person—up a ramp. Can you imagine how degrading that felt?! Not to mention the several times my chair fell backwards because somebody let go of me for a second. Inside the house was worse. My "room" was actually the living room. Life consisted of watching TV, sitting outside if it was warm, and possibly going to my outpatient therapy twice a week.

Rather than being the upgrade I had expected, living at home was hell! Every single night for years I begged God to take me, and every morning I woke up and ate my oatmeal, cussing God for making me go through another tedious, boring day. He did send me some angels though, in the form of my home health aides. They felt like my second moms, going above and beyond. In addition to taking care of my medical needs, they bought me Christmas presents and food and took me to the movies, the mall, and the hairdresser. Once one of my aides took me on vacation to the Smoky Mountains (close to forty-five minutes away from home) with her family.

Sometimes though, devils come disguised as angels. One of my aides told me God created my stroke because I had been a bad person. Not, I made some bad mistakes—I was, flat out, a bad person. I wanted to tell someone and get her fired, but it's not like my family or anybody was in the right frame of mind to hear my complaint. So, for the two years she worked with me, I was forced to pretend she didn't say that to me several times. Looking back, I should have told someone. My dilemma was that she knew my care and I didn't want to rock the boat for everybody else. Instead, I just dealt with it and nobody knew about what she said until after she quit.

As much as some of my family and friends apologized to me for not being there or putting me through that, part of me can't let go of that anger and hurt. And sadly, it still causes me to put up a shield with certain people. I don't think they understand how much they screwed me up mentally.

The first time Bre fed me after the stroke felt humiliating. Before my stroke, to save money and calories we sometimes bought one big dinner and split it. She went to dinner and saved me half of her chimichanga. As soon as she put the spoon to my mouth I started to cry uncontrollably. This was the girl I had driven to Daytona Beach with for Senior Week, made up stupid, silly "interpretive" dances to songs with, started college with, and now she had to feed me like a baby! I couldn't even look her in the eye, but I felt her fighting back the tears also. My best friend in the world! It felt awful. She must have told our friends about our experience, because none of them fed me for quite a while.

Although it was what I had hoped and prayed for, being home did not make all my dreams come true. It did, however, help me appreciate things more. The first time I got a shower and not a bed bath, I felt elated. And I was able to live with Blake again. We went to a few of his baseball games and every time Mom yelled, "Hit a homer for Sissy!" he delivered. I was also reunited with my dog, Harley. It was cute because loud noises scared Harley, and the second it thundered or somebody shot a gun (we lived down South with no close neighbors), Harley would run and jump on my lap.

Going through that all made me more grateful, but if you see anyone in that situation, please say something. It sucks.

19
What Lies Beneath

When you check out of the hospital, the nurse hands you all sorts of forms and pamphlets to help you adjust to life at home—lists of medications and when and how to take them, physical or occupational therapy exercises you must do, doctor's appointments you need to schedule, nutrition advice... But especially for us "extended stay" guests embarking on our "new lives," there are a lot of things they don't tell you. Whatever happened to common courtesy, folks? So I have taken the liberty of jotting down a few things you had better know after vamoosing the hospital with brand-new, full-body disabilities. Who knows, maybe they'll start passing this information out! You're welcome.

- You need to put your body on a schedule. Bathroom, eating, etc.
- You need to schedule everything around this body schedule.
- You can no longer eat what you want and when you want.
- Your body isn't your body anymore. Everybody sees you naked and grabs your ass to transfer you. Get over it!
- Go out in public even though you don't want to.
- People in public *and* some members of your family will treat you like a child, even though you are an intelligent adult!

- You get and deserve fabulous parking. You'll be incensed when you see people use it who *don't* need it.
- You need to learn to trust people with your body. You don't have to trust people with all things, but trust they will not let you get hurt or die.
- Things are no longer on your time. *Ever.*
- Always remember the sayings, "Don't bite the hand that feeds you" and "Don't judge a book by its cover."
- Suck up as much pain as possible.
- You just plain have to deal with *stupid shit* and ignorant comments all the time.
- These are the numbers you need to call... * insert important contacts*

I'm sure that there are a few other things that could be put down, but these are the main ones that I found important.

They also don't tell you that after a stroke or other neurological conditions, you get this issue called the pseudobulbar affect, also known as PBA. Ridiculous and embarrassing and annoying, it's uncontrollable crying and laughing—and everybody gets it. The crying part I accept and deal with. My family calls me Sappy Sue for my crying bursts. The laughing part, I swear up and down, "I did not have sexual relations with that woman" (Bill Clinton joke). To be clear, I did not develop that problem. Honestly, I must say I do sometimes laugh at inappropriate times, but I have a legit excuse. I do suffer from a nervous laugh; it's genetic from Mom. We both laugh when we get nervous or scared. Admitting the laughing part would be like having to admit I have another disability, and I'm not ready to accept that yet.

The first time I said, "Love you" to Blake, I smiled big, and then right before I cried, Blake said, "And...here comes Sappy Sue."

Allison, my former PT, read a post in my blog in which I complained about my PBA. She still worked at my rehabilitation center, and one of the doctors there suggested I try a relatively new medicine called Nudexta. That was nearly four years ago, and it works great! It doesn't stop me from being able to cry or laugh, but it helps a lot with the uncontrollable bursts. So that's a plus!

Another detail they don't tell you (males can skip this paragraph) is that after traumatic events your period usually stops for a few months. I didn't have one for close to six months. Mom kept saying, "lucky you," while I thought to myself, "That better be true, because I can't handle having a stroke and being pregnant."

They also don't tell you that most of your friends and some family take your sickness as unmanageable *for them* and choose to step back or out of your life. Never mind that you almost died and your whole world changed; it's all about them.

One big thing they don't tell you (on purpose, I think) is that, although you'll have lots of people helping you with daily activities, therapies, technology, and communication, you'll be taking a long emotional journey largely on your own. You have to learn to live your changes one by one and adjust to your new reality, growing and accepting that the former you is gone. But it's not all bad.

The "new" you is better and more understanding! You really don't know what you can handle until the shit hits the fan.

20
Kids Say the Darnedest Things

Comment from someone who knew me before my stroke: "Wow! You don't look like you used to!"

Well, no shit, Sherlock! But thank you for that keen, groundbreaking observation!

This chapter is dedicated to all the stupid, crazy, weird, annoying, and downright rude things people have said or done to me since I've appeared in public in designer disabilities. Trust me, it happens quite often. People do say the darnedest things. I assume they think they are nice, but they are in fact, rude. The fact that it needs its own chapter *should* alarm you.

I want to start by amending a statement I made earlier. In my Chapter 19 pamphlet I urged you to go out in public even when you don't want to, and while I stand by that, some days it's just not going to be possible. Some days you just want to hide in your house and avoid the BS that is attracted to someone in a wheelchair, and this is me telling you it's okay.

Now this is in no particular order, but trust me—each one is its individual version of *crazy*.

My favorite top 10 stupid questions, comments, and gestures:
1. The comment I opened this chapter with.
2. Do not pat me on the head like a dog. Just don't.

3. Just because I can't talk doesn't mean I'm hard of hearing. SO YOU DON'T HAVE TO YELL!
4. Don't talk babytalk to me and tickle my chin like I'm five years old.
5. "Since you can't move much you probably can't feel anything, right?" Umm, no, where did you get that? I can feel everything!
6. My name is not Jesse! It is Jessica or Jess.
7. "Don't hit her head. She already has enough brain damage."
8. "Just throw her around like a sack of potatoes."
9. If an adult or bratty child stares at me in public, I will almost always make a funny face back. A cute little curious kid gets a smile.
10. "Well, you must just be lazy all the time and not try hard."

That last one is the kicker! You can't make this stuff up. The first comment is one I hear all too often and it gets old, quick. I swear, if I earned a nickel for every time someone whispered or said that out loud to me, I would be able to live comfortably by now.

It's not like I haven't seen a mirror in fourteen years; I know what I look like. Not looking the same as my old self makes me shy now! I've joked about it with my friends and they always tell me it's not true and I look the same, but it's not as if I haven't heard the whispers: "Is that what she used to look like? How could somebody so pretty look like that now?" A nurse in Tennessee literally made that last comment, and she's damn lucky I didn't own my power chair yet. She would have been "accidentally" run over. Part of me wanted to smack her across the face and cuss her out, then the other part was saying to myself, *Just breathe, Jessica.*

Don't cry. Hearing crap like that hurts, but to the world I must act as if I didn't hear it and just smile. What they are in reality saying is, "Wow, you're ugly compared to how you used to look."

Something new is giving me my confidence back! I started it a few weeks ago, and it looks inappropriate, but it's strengthening my facial muscles and jawline. It's called a Jawzrcise. I put a special ball in my mouth and bite down, and it records twenty to forty pounds of pressure. I saw some slight differences, and then noticed a big difference compared to a photo of me from a few years ago. My face looks less round and more muscular. The Jawzrcise and somebody I know is helping me gain confidence

Can you believe that on several occasions somebody asked me, "How long are you?" Instead of, "How tall are you?" Really?! You want to get some measuring tape and measure me like a newborn baby? I'm 5 feet 9 inches *tall*, for your information. Technically, 5' 8½", so I round up. Sue me. What? In my family, and half my friends', my height is average-to-short. It's only since I've been able to stand that people gasp and say, "You're so tall!"

When I was younger my dream was to be six feet tall. Now that I'm wheelchair bound with limited mobility, my height is sometimes a complication (*Insert sappy violin music* for short people)—I'm too tall for this or that, I don't fit on my bed, sometimes I have to slouch in my chair for my communication device, and countless other inconveniences. Let's just say it's not easy.

One time a girl joked with me regarding my height, saying she wouldn't want to be my height because she wouldn't be able to put her hands up on her boyfriend's shoulders. Umm, it's not like I'm the attack of the fifty-foot woman. I'll have you know I have dated several guys taller than me, but guess what? It's a known fact that guys shorter than you are better in bed. It's the Napoleon complex, hello! So, who do you think wins in multiple aspects? Jessica-1, Naysayers-0.

Now, I've heard plenty of rude comments in my day. Some are from old friends, so it's easy to give them a smart-ass answer back. When they come from complete strangers, I must smile and think, *Will you just get the hell away from me please, weirdo?*

But these are a few more of my favorites to make you chuckle. I'll count backwards for comedic flair:

5. A stranger in a store walked up to me and said, "You are so cute; you must drive the boys crazy." Thanks, liar!

4. An old friend from high school said, "Well, you don't work as hard as me." So, you're saying I am lazy??

3. An old friend from high school told my friend: "Bless her heart, she was *normal* in high school."

2. Another old friend from high school said, "Well, it is good to see you smile in your pictures." To which I retorted, "Why wouldn't I be smiling?"

And the number one comment is from an old friend from work: "It is good you are doing as well as can be expected." Umm like, thank you, I think?

So, you've heard the crazy, weird, and rude; now here are the *annoying!*

Few things annoy me, but if they do, they thoroughly bother me. Some of the people I live with now yell and scream frequently and some of the others, along with some of the workers, *constantly complain* about it! I grew up with a little brother with ADHD and he loved to make repetitive noises. My nonverbal cousin with autism yells often, so the screaming doesn't bother me, but the constant complaining bugs the ever loving shit out of me!

Another secret annoyance of mine is able-bodied people complaining to me about being overweight. Seriously? You can get up and go walk around or go to the gym! People just complain to me about the stupidest stuff.

It makes me sad, though, when my friends talk about going to this bar or that gym and staying out until three a.m. Granted, I'm the grandma of my friends and conk out by ten or eleven p.m., but I would appreciate having the option. Little things like seeing a friend bring another friend a coffee to work "just because" gets to me. Bre used to bring breakfast to my work every day before graduating high school; I miss that.

You know what else? I hate seeing a kissing scene in a movie. Besides the fact that I'm probably sitting next to my mother, it makes me uncomfortable as hell. It also makes me pine for stuff like that. You don't know what you have 'til it's gone. I used to hold Mom's hand, inspecting each finger.

Every wrinkle and vein fascinated me. I really miss a guy touching the small of my back or brushing the hair off my neck to kiss it. And of course, tonsil hockey, haha!

Really, I just wish people would watch what they say and how they treat people. You never know how much it affects someone. Most times I am able to laugh it off, but that doesn't mean I find it funny.

21

Grownups

For the first few years after I came home from the hospital, everyone in my family felt depressed regarding me and other family issues. The house was awful for me. The state was taking away my home care, so my only option in Tennessee was a nursing home. Finally in 2009 Mom and I decided to move to Pennsylvania with Granny. It also seemed like the perfect chance for me to escape the stares and awkward encounters with people I used to know as friends and family.

It was my idea way back in 2004 to move in with Granny before Mom ever agreed to go. After my grandfather died Granny was lonely, so that helped the argument. And because of everything with Dad, my parents needed a break from each other.

It was a tougher decision for Blake. Before moving, Mom told Blake, "You're eighteen; it's your decision whether to move. But we are moving. You need one sane parent, and I am going insane here."

Blake told me recently, "At first it felt like you all were on vacation. Then it set in y'all were really gone."

Even though that breaks my heart, it was the greatest decision to move up here! The house was better for me (it had an actual ramp, haha) and my parents needed the little separation from each other to work on themselves, so it was much less stress for everybody.

From Granny's I attended daily rehab for about six months at a well-known facility in PA. Not really anything to write about there; it was uneventful (sorry if you know me and that offends you, but it's true and you probably know it).

In June of 2011 I finally moved out of Mom's (well, technically my grandmother's) house. Now I feel so old and mature, haha. Of course I love Mom and appreciate all she does for me, but things are different since my stroke. I was becoming too dependent on her for things I should have been learning to do myself. It's great to regain my independence! After begging Mom to allow me to live independently from her (for some reason I'm perpetually five in her eyes), I was finally able to move to an awesome facility in Delaware where I live today. For privacy's sake I am withholding the name but trust me, it's an awesome place!

My uncle, Austin's dad, suggested this place after Austin came to day camp here. Granny, Mom, my home health aide Jill, and I came for a tour and liked how it looked. Grudgingly, I do have to admit that the winning deal breaker for me was when one of the workers walked beside me and he was cute! Granted, it was a shallow deal breaker, but an important one. The application process normally takes two years or more, but mine was expedited once I started coming to exercise in their pool.

Before you live here you have to do some trial weekends, which they call respite stays. By the middle of the first respite I thought, *Holy shit! What was I thinking? Why did I let my hormones make such a big decision? I hate this place.* Because I don't talk, I got frustrated when the staff didn't know my preferences (for example, needing the sensor on my nose for my Dynavox or brushing my teeth *after* breakfast). It was hard at first, but now that I live here and they all know me and I know them, I enjoy it.

What I love most about this place is that they treat me as though the chair *doesn't* exist. If I want to do some activity, like going to a museum, ninety percent of the time they figure out a way to make it happen. The staff actually suggested I go snow tubing and set everything up. I go every February and it's the best day *ever*. If I need to go to the store or hear of a fun concert, we email back and forth and they schedule it. When I first moved here I wanted Mom to go to every doctor appointment with me. Now I'm like, "I got this myself!"

> The first time I went snow tubing, I cried like a little kid when it was time to leave. I was so grateful to be given the opportunity to have so much fun and just appreciated every minute. When was the last time you were overwhelmed with gratitude? And how did you react?

Of course, some things and people here do make me mad. For example, the communication between departments is not good—sometimes they treat us like children (requiring "permission"), and everything is soooo slow most of the time (for me to get Listerine the first time took a week). All in all, I can't complain. Fact of the matter is, my home is good. I'm afforded opportunities that most people with disabilities don't have the privilege of experiencing, so for that I am thankful. Knowing how few places can provide the necessary level of care, we are *damn* lucky! It's about the journey and the steps I am taking to find myself again. In helping me do that, this place will forever be a part of me, as will the people I have met.

Being here, I don't have to have somebody grabbing my hand off my driving handle if I get too close, somebody looking over my shoulder, somebody calling my friends to "babysit" me...the list could go on and on. I am proud to say that last year, I got a credit card! It doesn't have much of a limit, but it's helping me establish credit. Gaining my financial independence feels incredible! The first time Mom and I went to the store and I paid for everything, I almost cried. It was my proudest moment in years! Some purchases still require Mommy's money, but luckily not many. This woman is empowered!

22
To Hell and Back

In their hit song "Wide Open Spaces," country group The Dixie Chicks sang about finding your own life and your own dreams. Now that I'm no longer under my parents' roof, I feel like I'm living my own version of that song.

"Would you ever move back home?" a friend asked.

"Hell no!" I responded. Mom couldn't do half the physical, occupational, speech, and other therapies I get here. Not to mention all the physical and psychological independence I have gained living "independently."

A typical day in my life now looks like this:

Time	Monday	Tuesday	Wednesday	Thursday	Friday
9 AM	Breakfast	Breakfast	Breakfast	Breakfast	Breakfast
10 AM	Therapy	Homework	Homework	Therapy	Therapy
Noon	Lunch	Lunch	Lunch	Lunch	Lunch
1 PM	Homework	Therapy	Therapy	Therapy	Homework
5 PM	Dinner	Dinner	Dinner	Dinner	Dinner
6 PM	Computer	Computer	Computer	Computer	Computer
10 PM	Bed	Bed	Bed	Bed	Bed

Therapies range from physical to aquatic to massage. Yes, I said *massage*. Jealous? Once or twice a week I get an hour-long full-body massage. It feels soooo good. The masseuse rubs all my sore muscles. You can bend and stretch whenever. Although I am capable, I can't move whenever I want the same way as you. For me to stretch, somebody must remove my wheelchair tray and Dynavox so I can bend down.

A couple of times a year, students from a Disability Studies class at a local university come. Some of the students interview me and I give them one of my speeches on my life and stroke. Then they turn it into a presentation.

It's like a fulltime job living here through the week. Weekends I finally get to rest unless I have homework. If I actually have free time I chat with friends, watch TV, surf the internet, and study for class. The game Mahjong is my Zen moment. When people say I am lazy, I laugh. Like, seriously? You have no idea.

The chair I sit on in the shower has a big hole in the bottom so my aides can wash my butt and stuff. I try so hard not to laugh. Not because it feels good, but because that scene plays in my head from the movie *Father of the Bride 2*, when they mistakenly take Steve Martin to the proctology exam and he *runs out, saying, "Excu-u-use me! Do I know you?"*

Over the past couple of years I have achieved some true milestones. I can help with some of my bathing and feeding, and my speech therapist programmed the center's elevator codes into my Dynavox so I can go downstairs by myself. Using one of my "MacGyver moves" (that's what I call my weird, thinking-outside-the-box moves), I can open my bedroom door. First I pull up close with the door on my right. Then I lift my arm, get the handle in between my knuckles, and push down. Most of the time my hands stay clenched in a fist, so if you *give me a minute* I can try a "MacGyver move." I hate it when people don't let me try!

What's my best "MacGyver move"? Feeding myself doesn't really qualify. The OTs here where I live already owned the device. It's just an IV pole with a spring and slings for my elbow and wrist. I push down to scoop the food, and then the spring bounces my arm up to reach my mouth. It's messy and I usually drop food everywhere, but worth the mess to do it myself.

When I first learned to drive my wheelchair, numerous therapists told me, "You *can't* drive with your hand; you can probably only drive with switches." Boiling with fury I thought, *I survived a massive brain stem stroke. I should not be alive, and you are going to tell me what I am capable of? Oh, hell, no! Watch me prove you wrong.* Fast forward a few years (well, past the year of recovery described in Chapter 6), and now I *do* drive with my hand. To hear the word "CAN'T" remains my best motivation because that word pisses me off!! What's the one word that infuriates you?

To be able to do that stuff now is great, but part of me thinks, *Whoopty friggin' doo, it's not much, really. It's not like I have complete independence.* I know you're thinking, *quit complaining, Jessica! At least it's something.*

One factor (of many) about my stroke that bothers me is that my right side is stronger than my left. I used to be left-handed, but for now (until my left arm gets stronger) I have to do things right-handed. And let me tell you—relearning to write and switching your dominant hand is not easy! My legs remain a different story because I tend to overcompensate for my left side's retardation (the medical word, not the mean, derogatory word). I can bear most of my weight now while standing and when I physically take steps I walk better with my left leg. My body is just weird now. Even my old PT, Allison, joked: "Your body is weird." When I studied the brain for my psychology class I finally understood what she meant. My stroke should have affected the right side more since I used to be left-dominant, but it decided to do the opposite.

  The physical and psychological independence I talked about earlier is fabulous! I feel like a real woman in my thirties. Therefore, I embrace every birthday now and have earned every wrinkle and grey hair—but thankfully, none yet, haha!
  A line in "Wide Open Spaces" says, "She needs new faces." I needed new people and friends to see and understand and help the "new" me achieve my goals.

23
A Walk to Remember

Strength is a mysterious force. You can't see it or hear it. You can't even feel it most of the time. But it magically appears—filling your entire being—when you need it most.

When my stroke first happened, I was at my weakest physically, emotionally, and spiritually. I cried constantly and spelled "why" by blinking to Mom and my friend AJ. Mom, Dad, and Granny tried to explain what happened to me, but I don't think even they understood yet. "You're sick," Mom kept saying. "You don't have cancer or anything, but you're sick."

That was the most confusing and heartbreaking news. I was a nineteen-year-old girl with her whole life in front of her! Caught between life and death, it just wasn't fair. Why did this happen to me? *Like seriously, why? I am just a normal teenaged girl. Everybody takes birth control.* Was this karma? Was I a bad person?

For many years after my stroke I was furious with God. Finally, I was getting the perfect life and then He decided to pull the rug from under me. It wasn't until I started studying my stroke that I realized, *Wow! He really loves me. I should be dead. By some dumb luck I am among the two percent to survive brain stem strokes?*

Now I see it more like, why not me? God picked me, *little ol' Jessica Davenport,* a southern redneck from slow-paced, beautiful East Tennessee. I could have died, but His will always makes a way. It's the only way I can explain a blood clot forming somewhere in my body and traveling to my heart—which, incidentally, has a patent foramen ovale, allowing the clot to go through to my brainstem and cause a stroke.

We knew nothing about the hole in my heart. All those years I played sports and underwent many physical examinations, and nobody heard anything abnormal. The clot's voyage doesn't sound like a good thing, but had it stayed in my heart I could have died. While I can complain about what went wrong, I'd be ignoring what went right. That hole in my heart happened to be a "stroke of luck," no pun intended. Seems like He picked the perfect girl with a loud mouth to spread the knowledge of the possible dangers of birth control. And who am I to reject that mission?

It's all a gift from the Man upstairs. You might not see it, but I do. For all the "What ifs" of my stroke, you must admit it's amazing I'm still here! God could have taken me home like so many other sweet girls with my disorder, but He picked me to stick around. Since He let me live and remain of sound mind, you are going to listen to this big mouth talk and educate people about the dangers of birth control until the day I die. I know those girls who got to go home to heaven would have done the same for me! They say God can decide how to humble you, and this truly and positively humbled me. Despite being physically weak in many ways, spiritually I'm gaining strength every day.

In my heart, I believe God lets bad things happen sometimes for a reason. I love Him, but I do have a torn relationship with Him. Part of me is angry that He let this dreadful thing happen, but I'm honored He picked me. Major contradiction. Why the hell me? *What is so damn special about me?* Is it that I'm a big mouth and I feel the need to educate people? My guess is that He probably put that on my heart. This passion wasn't there before, I don't think. Thousands of other girls died from strokes or embolisms due to this disorder and this deadly combination. Why didn't He pick them to live instead of me? Despite all my questions, I'm glad He let me stay. My biggest question is, why? Does He love me more to let me continue living or does He love them more because He let them go to heaven? I guess I won't know the answer until I get there. But I want to know now! *Well? Answer me, dammit!*

No answer yet.

Honestly, I don't think I'll ever get my answer, but there remains one point I'm sure of. I am so thankful this stroke happened! It taught me so much about everything, everyone, and myself. God wouldn't bring you to it if He couldn't pull you through it. Yep, I'm one tough bi-otch! I never knew I possessed such reserves of strength, or that of course it was because God guided me ("pulled me through it") that I was able to access them. I have lived through a lot since March 17, 2004, which you all know now is the day I had my stroke. If you're given the choice to have your life change completely, take it. You learn a lot!

A few months ago, I got a tattoo on my left upper inner arm that says, "God wouldn't bring you to it if He couldn't pull you through it" in black cursive with "God" and "He" highlighted in green. The green is for this book and my blog. Coincidentally, the tattoo artist had only two green dyes, and one happened to be the exact hue of green I needed.

Dear God, could you maybe give me a break on the emotional strength for a while and focus on some other strength? haha.

24
Love and Marriage

I don't know that I could ever fall in love in this body. They say you can't love someone else until you love yourself, and sadly but truthfully, I don't love myself in this *different* body. Don't get me wrong—I like myself, but I don't love every single aspect of myself. I am trying to learn, but it's a gradual process!

How could I write a chapter on love without talking about Trav? It would be foolish to say I was "in love" with him, but I can't deny that I loved him. Until writing this book, I didn't realize how much I loved Trav. What we had felt different from anything else I'd experienced. We had known each other since middle school but didn't become best friends until our junior year of high school.

We always joked that we were like an engaged couple *without* the sex. I believe I loved Trav so much because he was the only man I didn't need to sleep with for him to like me. Attending the parent meetings for Blake's baseball team, the joke between us was that Blake was our adopted son. We said, "I love you" to each other constantly, so I thought it was real, but apparently not. He's gay now, so my lighthearted twist on the situation (to make me feel better) is that he must have used me as his "beard." He was always gay, but I didn't notice it—well, I probably chose not to notice.

Bre came to my house the night Trav came out. We both laughed: "Duh, it was so obvious!" But I cried to myself, thinking, So it wasn't real? Am I that blind? I joke about being his beard and avoid telling you that I stay up crying some nights thinking about what we had. Earlier I told you I developed feelings for him; mine were real, but were his? For some reason, he didn't tell me for years that he was gay.

I have only been in love, lustful love, once and it just so happened that I didn't realize my feelings until right after my stroke. So, I guess neither of my loves counts.

Honestly, it scares the shit out of me to say that I want to be in love, to give my whole heart to someone else, no questions asked... Sometimes I still feel like that girl with teenage insecurities involving love. My dating experience remained cryogenically frozen while my body aged. I have to remind myself, *Come on, Jessica, you're over thirty. It's time to think about marriage and kids!* Is a relationship still possible for me? Logistically? Physically?

Ever since I was little, motherhood has been my dream. Now because of my stroke and blood disorder, I don't know if that's possible anymore. My blood disorder, Prothrombin 20210, is genetic, but we still don't know from which side of my family it originates. Hold on, let me get my lab coat and explain this better.

When you are conceived you get twenty-three chromosomes from each parent. Within the chromosomes are genes; within genes are alleles. Homozygous alleles are from both parents and a heterozygous allele is from one parent. For example, eye color's an allele. My mom and dad both have brown eyes, creating two homozygous alleles, giving my brother brown eyes.

My blood disorder is a genotype (set of genes) that is heterozygous, from one parent. So until Mom or my biological father gets tested, I remain SOL. In a brochure on *Prothrombin Gene Mutation* from the University of Iowa, Dr. Steven Lentz, Director of the Division of Hematology, Oncology, and Blood & Marrow Transplantation at the University of Iowa Health Care's Carver College of Medicine, writes, "People with one copy of this gene have about a five times greater chance of getting a blood clot than someone without the prothrombin gene change."[17] The blood disorder most likely isn't detrimental to Blake or my two sisters and brother from my biological dad since most people with the disorder don't ever develop a clot. I was just the "lucky" one of my siblings.

Researching my blood disorder has given me insecurities since it causes so many gynecological and fertility issues. If I get pregnant I run the risk of developing another clot, as well as miscarriage, stillbirth, and preeclampsia (high blood pressure all through pregnancy).[18] I don't want to be mad at God. But it's like, *What else can you throw at me?* Of course, there are other options and avenues such as adoption and surrogacy, but should they let somebody with my physical issues adopt a child? Who knows? Probably not. And that petrifies the hell out of me! This sounds selfish, but I want a little me with my mannerisms and looks. I want to hold my baby and hear some stranger compliment me, saying, "He is adorable!" or "She looks just like you."

Right now, I try to remind myself, *Just sit back and go for the ride.*

Reading about my blood disorder is like checking items off a list—except these were all things I had been doing:
1. *Don't smoke*
2. *Don't take birth control*
3. *Don't drink excessively*

Kids stay front and center in my dreams and marriage is an unknown bonus for me. Right now, God's the only man singing to me: "Girl, you're amazing, just the way you are."

It's almost comical, me wanting kids so much. It makes me chuckle, now that I think of it. That is a lot of pressure to put on a kid: "Mommy survived a stroke and overcame its debilitating effects for you." I still want kids, but poor things, haha! I guess we will just see how my deck deals!

Honestly, I just don't see who would want someone like me. Well, at least someone I'm attracted to too. Plenty of guys hit on me now (usually creeps); I'm just not attracted to them. In case you can't tell, the perfectionist in me remains hard on myself. I guess that bulimic girl must still be buried in me saying, "You're not good enough." People now tell me how cute I am, and my immediate reaction is thinking, *Haha, you're being nice*. From some people, I accept the compliment; others are just being nice. I was and will always stay obsessed with my weight. And I never thought I was outstandingly cute. But now I look back at pictures of me and think, *Damn! Look at that skinny hottie, haha! My mom and biological father sure made a pretty baby!*

My biological dad's kids and I look soooo much alike. We all video chat sometimes, and OMG...my youngest sister—it's like looking in a mirror before my stroke.

This stroke took so much away from me. However, in return for what I lost, I gained in people and places and experiences. Because of what I've lived through, I am a better woman, so for that I remain thankful. Besides, in a way I enjoy my "celibacy" (I use the quotations only because I didn't *choose* my celibacy). I have gotten and am getting to know myself more and what I want my future husband to be like:

1. He's gotta make me laugh.
2. He needs some Faith.
3. A good head on his shoulders.
4. Patience!
5. I usually say to my girls, he must be kind of strong to pick me up lol!

I still think about sex sometimes and miss it. The thought of being naked in this post-stroke body in front of somebody else (and they're not a caregiver) turns my stomach though. One time I met this guy and I thought we flirted. Then later that evening he rejected me, and it turned into two hours of me sobbing. Trying to tell one of my aides, it took twenty minutes for me to type between sobs, "My (gasp) post-stroke (gasp) insecurity (gasp) is real. Nobody (gasp) will ever (gasp) love me. I am just (gasp) ugly."

But then again that whole panic attack reminds me of the panic attack with Bre when we first moved to college. That turned out okay in the long run, so maybe this will too. Maybe I should get back out there and put money where my mouth is. Continuously now, I try to remind myself, *Quit being a control freak. Sit back, Jessica, and let "Jesus take the wheel" on marriage and kids. Just do you, Boo. Be the best you, whatever your body.*

I don't believe I am the best me yet. But I'm working hard to expand my vision beyond the physical manifestation of who I am. Focusing on my own physical perfection is my main deterrent. Inside, I feel sexy as shit. I say to myself, *You are a badass mofo, you survived a brainstem stroke, you write a blog, you wrote a book, you go to college—and that list could go on and on.* (Lord, help my potty mouth next, haha!)

25
Back to School

What's the best way to stop obsessing over yourself? Help others. I did.

Deciding to educate people regarding the possible dangers of birth control is easy for me now, but when my stroke first happened everyone needed to adapt to our "new normal." I was so busy comprehending it all, I didn't have time or energy for anything—or anyone—else. This sounds selfish, but teaching other people something I didn't truthfully understand myself was out of the question.

In 2010, I stopped worrying about me and started my blog and my other forms of social media! All my social media websites are so important to me—they are my babies (the real ones will come someday). I started my blog, www.jessbsstroke.com, not only to talk to my family and friends about my accomplishments and hardships, but also to educate people I don't know all over the world about my stroke and the dangers of birth control.

Honestly, my blog started from boredom. Back then I lived with Mom and Granny, having moved to Pennsylvania from Tennessee, and was between rehabilitation therapy centers. I told Mom and my home health aide Jill that I felt bored and wanted a job. Being a busybody is normal for me; I can't sit still for long. I get it from Granny. Instead of a regular nine-to-five job, they both suggested I start a blog.

Coincidentally, I had been thinking for some time about starting a blog about my stroke. My friend Lisa (from the wedding I was supposed to be in) showed me her family's blog, and it looked easy enough. I guess I just needed a kick in the ass to finally just do it. Jill started the blog for me and said, "Here, finish it." Neither of us knew what it would become. Now it has thousands of views across the country and around the world! The social media pages were all me, though—I just linked most of what I had to my blog. Nothing special.

Roughly two years ago I rejoined the outside world and was blessed with a full scholarship to Wilmington University in New Castle, Delaware! My major is Health Science, and I'm also working toward a Certificate in Digital Marketing. Becoming a birth control counselor or educator (my dream job!) and helping women decide which birth control is right for them are my top priorities now. It fills me with honor and excitement when friends or strangers ask *me* for birth control advice!

Going back to school after such a long break is difficult for anybody, but embarking on this journey with a disability is a thousand times more difficult! Writing a paper takes me at least a week: I must format it correctly and type each character one at a time—no touch typing for me (*sad face emoji*). When I first started back to school, I spent several days crying in frustration to my family and friends: "In the time it takes you to type a page, I can only type four sentences!"

But I am keeping up with my classmates and look forward to each new course. My biggest gripe—some people belittle my collegiate skills! It's like that scene in the movie *Legally Blonde* in which Elle's ex accuses her of not being smart. And like Elle, I have a thing or two to show everyone!

26
Easy A

I am not a doctor and don't think I'll ever be, so there are parts of this chapter that are from the internet. Even after reading this, you should still talk to your doctor to decide what kind of birth control is right for you. What kind of doctor, you ask? Well, you probably don't want to ask your podiatrist (foot doctor) concerning your vagina and birth control. Your best bet is your gynecologist or family practice physician. I may not be the brightest bulb in the tanning bed, but I have lived with this for several years and know a thing or two. So now it's time to get to the boring (Did I say that?), but *very* important medical information side of my story. Put your thinking cap on.

Let me first begin by explaining hormones and their purpose. Hormones are chemical substances in our bodies made by our endocrine glands to help specific organs. Everyone makes their own hormones, but sometimes not enough. When you are deficient in a hormone, the doctor usually has you take medication with that hormone to balance everything out. Sometimes this medication is beneficial, but in other cases it isn't. Adding other substances (like some types of birth control) that contain hormones can upset the delicate balance and damage your organs or cause malfunctions. According to Planned Parenthood, hormones in birth control make women more vulnerable to "heart attack, stroke, blood clots, and liver tumors."[19]

I always tell my friends and anybody who will listen to use *non-hormonal* birth control. Some examples would include condoms, diaphragms, sponges, and copper IUDs. A copper IUD with a condom is my recommendation; the IUD just stays in your body for ten years, and you don't have to remember to take a pill every day. Even though I suggest the copper IUD, it isn't for everybody. Your healthcare provider will discourage use if you're allergic to metal or have uterine abnormalities that interfere with the placement of the IUD.[20]

This is probably TMI, but I already opened up enough to you in this book, so what's a little more gonna hurt? I used to always make the guy wear a condom even though I was on birth control. So there, I'm sticking to my suggestion: use a condom and some other kind of birth control. Besides, condoms reduce the chance of spreading STDs and HIV. Non-hormonal birth control may not be one hundred percent effective like birth control with hormones, but it is safer. And you can't put a price on safety.

If you don't like my suggestion of non-hormonal birth control, at least try a low-estrogen or progestin-only birth control. These don't mess with your own hormones quite as much. Your doctor should help you decide. And don't be scared to ask your doctor questions!

My blood disorder isn't the only genetic thrombophilia-type blood disorder (disorders that make you form clots more than normal). According to the University of Iowa Health Care, these also include:
- Factor V Leiden
- Protein C deficiency
- Protein S deficiency
- Antithrombin deficiency[21]

Some doctors may disagree with my no hormones suggestion, so ask for a blood test called a coagulation panel. It tests to see if you clot easily. Blood clots can be detrimental or life threatening if not recognized early. Dr.

Steven Lentz writes, "Things that may trigger or cause blood clots to form include: surgery, trauma (injury) or fractures, bed rest or sitting or lying still for several hours at a time, cancer and chemotherapy, intravenous catheters, estrogen use, pregnancy, or air travel."[22]

Once you get your blood tested you will know for sure *if* you are able to safely take hormones and which ones. For example, because of my blood disorder I can't take estrogen. If doctors had checked my blood, they wouldn't have allowed me to switch to the ring because it contains progestin and estrogen. I'm just thankful for the huge variety of birth control types these days, non-hormonal or hormonal (estrogen or progestin). The list is huge!

When you talk to your doctor, know your shit! Even the FDA website tells you to know shit (aka options) before you talk to your healthcare provider. It saddens and infuriates me when people don't heed my warnings. Imagine me standing in front of you shaking your shoulders, crying and screaming, "Don't be like me, dammit! Educate yourself before starting birth control." After you read this book and my blog (www.jessbsstroke.com) go check out other websites on the possible dangers of birth control. Two of my favorite websites are www.informedchoiceforeamerika.com and www.hormonesmatter.com. And make sure you visit Planned Parenthood's website, www.plannedparenthood.org, where you can download an app to track your period. It also provides customized appointment reminders and puts birth control and sexual health resources from the experts at Planned Parenthood at your fingertips.

I'm not a doctor, and don't play one on TV. But my personal experience and research have earned me a degree in frankness. I must share what I know. Do your own research and ask your doctor lots of questions about hormones, blood clots, and all of your options before choosing a method of birth control.

27
A Fork in the Road

Life doesn't stop for anyone. Physically and mentally I'm over thirty, yet part of me still feels like that little nineteen-year-old girl. I reckon I skipped my twenties and everything is coming back to me in my thirties.

When I say this to Laci (whom I have known since way before my stroke) and other friends my age, they just say, "Oh, it's okay, you didn't miss anything." But to tell the truth, I missed a decade of my life. The twenties are when you establish yourself financially, mentally, sexually. You get your shit together. And I have none of that stuff established yet. People around me talk about buying cars, houses—yet I can barely buy a high-quality jacket.

One day my friend AJ gossiped about our friends and explained to me that, at twenty-two (his age at the time), "I would rather, like most people our age, hold off on sex until we establish the relationship. And not just jump into bed like you did." It's harsh, but true! I did used to do that. Yeah, my twenties got taken from me.

Everyone my age is getting great jobs, finding their soul mates, getting married and having babies, and I'm just sitting here in my wheelchair with my blog and this book. While I am happy for them, I can't help but want more. I just feel so out of touch with everything that is going on in the outside world. Is it wrong to want more?

When I was younger I was petrified of turning thirty. I mean, who isn't? Now I love being over 30! You have read throughout this book how much of a planner and perfectionist I am, but I see now that you *can't* plan everything. Since my stroke, I am ecstatic to be out of my crappy twenties and in a new decade! I earned every age milestone I achieved!

When my time in the first rehab was coming to an end, my speech therapist took Mom and me upstairs to the computer lab so I could communicate with her (and, in all honesty, discuss the menu I wanted after months of hospital food). It was the short period of time before my communication device, so I took the opportunity to say something more than yes or no.

My therapist asked, "What do you want more than anything?" I knew she meant, what *food.*

I simply said, "To be normal."

Neither Mom nor my therapist knew how to respond. Maybe it was out of place for me to express my feelings at that moment, but I jumped at my opportunity. To blend into a crowd would be a true gift from God. I want to go out in public and have people *not* stare at me. Mom makes a joke of the public stares now though, whispering to me, "Everybody's staring at us. This must be what a celebrity feels like."

Even though big crowds scare the *shit* out of me, I genuinely enjoy getting to do speaking engagements to tell my story and educate people about the possible dangers of birth control. I get nervous and shake before the speeches, so if Mom's there she always says, "You are fine. Besides, it's your Dynavox talking, not you." Plus, she and Dad didn't raise me to be scared and not try something.

Several people have asked me, "How do you stay so strong?" My quick response would be my faith, but my long and tangible answer would be how my parents raised us: You try it no matter what, because you might enjoy it after.

As a child, I cried while standing in line with my parents for a roller coaster. I thought it was going to be scary, but it turned out to be crazy exciting! Every parent reading this is probably flabbergasted they made us cry trying something, but it made my brother and me independent and willing to try anything!

I'm over thirty, and I still live like that. From public speaking to sitting on the edge of the physical therapy mat, to surfing—all things that scare the *bejesus* out of me—the feeling of accomplishment afterward makes it all worth it! It's like drinking five cups of strong coffee. Yeah, I would say my children and probably my brother's children will be raised just like that. Try it, no matter what—because you might love it.

I guess my little spiel alluded to the fact that I still use my Dynavox to talk. Although I can say a few one-syllable words sometimes, my speech is not substantial...yet. Quite frankly, I'm not ready to give up on trying. That is the main point I've learned through all this, and something I want each of you readers to remember— you never, ever, ever give up on yourself. No matter what people say or think—NEVER!

Even though I'm accomplishing something new all the time, I still dream of achieving more. A friend once asked me, "What are your dreams?" Honestly, my dreams are probably stupid and mundane to you. I dream of pushing the elevator button myself, of holding the TV remote in my hand and changing the channel by myself; no more having the freaking commands for them programmed into my Dynavox. I want to flip the bird to a jerk and not have somebody jokingly do it for me. Put both of my arms around a friend and both of us squeezing each other equally chest to chest (bet you never thought of a hug so technically). Stand up and dance with my brother at each of our weddings. Okay, so neither of us is engaged, but it's going to happen someday! I dream of the day my brother's and my kids play together at Christmas as we did with our cousins. Truly talking to a friend on the phone stays one of my biggest dreams.

Slowly but surely, I'm accomplishing my dreams and it is amazing because, even a few years ago, I didn't know if any of them was possible. You dream of these things, and don't really know if they are going to happen. It's just crazy that everything is coming true! I feel like I'm healing from the inside out. When I learn more about myself and spread the word about my stroke and the dangers of birth control I somehow do better physically.

My name is Jessica Davenport, and I approve this message.

The End.
Well not really, but you know what I mean.

Notes

1. "CT Scan," Mayo Clinic, Accessed May 9, 2018. https://www.mayoclinic.org/tests-procedures/ct-scan/about/pac-20393675.

2. "Lumbar Puncture (LP)," Johns Hopkins Medicine, Accessed May 12, 2018. https://www.hopkinsmedicine.org/healthlibrary/test_procedures/neurological/lumbar_puncture_92,P07666.

3. "Friend," Merriam-Webster, Accessed May 14, 2018. https://www.merriam-webster.com/dictionary/friend.

4. Satoshi Kanazawa, "Why Intelligent People Use More Drugs," *Psychology Today,* Nov. 1, 2010. https://www.psychologytoday.com/us/blog/the-scientific-fundamentalist/201011/why-intelligent-people-use-more-drugs.

5. "Friend," Urban Dictionary, Accessed May 15, 2018. https://www.urbandictionary.com/define.php?term=friends.

6. "Coma," Mayo Clinic, Accessed May 5, 2018. https://www.mayoclinic.org/diseases-conditions/coma/symptoms-causes/syc-20371099.

7. "Characteristics of a Near-Death Experience," IANDS, Accessed May 27, 2018. https://www.iands.org/ndes/about-ndes/characteristics.html.

8. Christopher L. Heffner, "Chapter 2: Section 3: The Brain and Nervous System," AllPsych, Accessed May 2, 2018. https://allpsych.com/psychology101/brain/.

9. "Prothrombin Thrombophilia," NIH Library of Medicine, Accessed May 1, 2018. https://ghr.nlm.nih.gov/condition/prothrombin-thrombophilia#statistics.

10. "Patent Foramen Ovale (PFO)," American Heart Association, Accessed May 1, 2018. http://www.heart.org/HEARTORG/Conditions/More/CardiovascularConditionsofChildhood/Patent-Foramen-Ovale-PFO_UCM_469590_Article.jsp#.WvtNLy8-LLg.

11. "Pulmonary Embolism," Healthline, Accessed April 30, 2018. https://www.healthline.com/health/pulmonary-embolus#symptoms.

12. *Christian's Story Part 1: Surviving Brain Stem Stroke,* American Heart Association Midwest, Video 4:35, Published June 27, 2016. https://www.youtube.com/watch?v=CaVxRG6_UBA.

13. "Brain Stem," Stroke Network, Accessed May 17, 2018. http://www.strokeeducation.info/brain/brainstem/index.htm.

14. "Coma," Mayo Clinic.

15. "Tracheostomy Service," Johns Hopkins Medicine, Accessed May 18, 2018. https://www.hopkinsmedicine.org/tracheostomy/about/what.html.

16. "As your life changes, so will your circle," Quotefinity, Pinterest, Accessed May 27, 2018. https://www.pinterest.com/offsite/?token=660-602&url=https%3A%2F%2Fwww.instagram.com%2Fp%2FBgjQslalxQc%2F&pin=664492119994276015&client_tracking_params=CwABAAAADDM1MDg2NDQyMjQ5MQA.

17. "Thrombophilia: Information for Patients," University of Iowa Health Care, Accessed May 4, 2018. https://www.healthcare.uiowa.edu/labs/lentz/Information_For_Patients/PDF/Prothrombin%20Gene%20Mutation%20Brochure.pdf.

18. "The Risks of Prothrombin Gene Mutation in Pregnancy," Healthline, Accessed May 2, 2018. https://www.healthline.com/health/pregnancy/prothrombin-gene-mutation#3.

19. "How Safe is the Birth Control Pill?" Planned Parenthood, Accessed May 6, 2018. https://www.plannedparenthood.org/learn/birth-control/birth-control-pill/how-safe-is-the-birth-control-pill.

20. "ParaGard (copper IUD)," Mayo Clinic, Accessed May 14, 2018. https://www.mayoclinic.org/tests-procedures/paragard/about/pac-20391270.

21. "Thrombophilia: Information for Patients," University of Iowa Health Care.

22. Ibid.

Bibliography

"As your life changes, so will your circle." Quotefinity. Pinterest. Accessed May 27, 2018. https://www.pinterest.com/offsite/?token=660-602&url=https%3A%2F%2Fwww.instagram.com%2Fp%2FBgjQslalxQc%2F&pin=664492119994276015&client_tracking_params=CwABAAAADDM1MDg2NDQyMjQ5MQA.

"Brain Stem." Stroke Network. Accessed May 17, 2018. http://www.strokeeducation.info/brain/brainstem/index.htm.

"Characteristics of a Near-Death Experience." IANDS. Accessed May 27, 2018. https://www.iands.org/ndes/about-ndes/characteristics.html.

Christian's Story Part 1: Surviving Brain Stem Stroke. American Heart Association Midwest. Video 4:35. Published June 27, 2016. https://www.youtube.com/watch?v=CaVxRG6_UBA.

"Coma." Mayo Clinic. Accessed May 5, 2018. https://www.mayoclinic.org/diseases-conditions/coma/symptoms-causes/syc-20371099.

"CT Scan." Mayo Clinic. Accessed May 9, 2018. https://www.mayoclinic.org/tests-procedures/ct-scan/about/pac-20393675.

"Friend." Merriam-Webster. Accessed May 14, 2018. https://www.merriam-webster.com/dictionary/friend.

"Friend." Urban Dictionary. Accessed May 15, 2018. https://www.urbandictionary.com/define.php?term=friends.

Heffner, Christopher L. "Chapter 2: Section 3: The Brain and Nervous System." AllPsych. Accessed May 2, 2018. https://allpsych.com/psychology101/brain/.

"How Safe is the Birth Control Pill?" Planned Parenthood. Accessed May 6, 2018. https://www.plannedparenthood.org/learn/birth-control/birth-control-pill/how-safe-is-the-birth-control-pill.

Kanazawa, Satoshi. "Why Intelligent People Use More Drugs." *Psychology Today,* Nov. 1, 2010. https://www.psychologytoday.com/us/blog/the-scientific-fundamentalist/201011/why-intelligent-people-use-more-drugs.

"Lumbar Puncture (LP)." Johns Hopkins Medicine. Accessed May 12, 2018. https://www.hopkinsmedicine.org/healthlibrary/test_procedures/neurological/lumbar_puncture_92,P07666.

"ParaGard (copper IUD)." Mayo Clinic. Accessed May 14, 2018. https://www.mayoclinic.org/tests-procedures/paragard/about/pac-20391270.

"Patent Foramen Ovale (PFO)." American Heart Association. Accessed May 1, 2018. http://www.heart.org/HEARTORG/Conditions/More/CardiovascularConditionsofChildhood/Patent-Foramen-Ovale-PFO_UCM_469590_Article.jsp#.WvtNLy8-LLg.

"Prothrombin Thrombophilia." NIH Library of Medicine. Accessed May 1, 2018. https://ghr.nlm.nih.gov/condition/prothrombin-thrombophilia#statistics.

"Pulmonary Embolism." Healthline. Accessed April 30, 2018. https://www.healthline.com/health/pulmonary-embolus#symptoms.

"The Risks of Prothrombin Gene Mutation in Pregnancy." Healthline. Accessed May 2, 2018. https://www.healthline.com/health/pregnancy/prothrombin-gene-mutation#3.

"Thrombophilia: Information for Patients." University of Iowa Health Care. Accessed May 4, 2018. https://www.healthcare.uiowa.edu/labs/lentz/Information_For_Patients/PDF/Prothrombin%20Gene%20Mutation%20Brochure.pdf.

"Tracheostomy Service." Johns Hopkins Medicine. Accessed May 18, 2018.

https://www.hopkinsmedicine.org/tracheostomy/about/what.html.

www.ingramcontent.com/pod-product-compliance
Lightning Source LLC
Chambersburg PA
CBHW071056240526
45471CB00016B/1966